# Ministering to Minds Diseased

## A history of psychiatric treatment

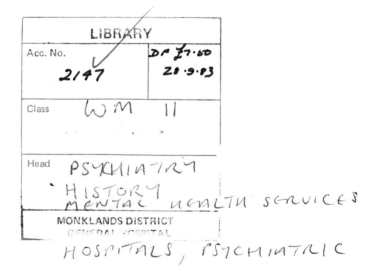

Canst thou not minister to a mind diseas'd;
Pluck from the memory a rooted sorrow;
Raze out the written troubles of the brain;
And with some sweet oblivious antidote
Cleanse the stuff'd bosom of the perilous stuff
Which weighs upon the heart?

*Macbeth*

# Ministering to
# MINDS DISEASED

## A HISTORY OF PSYCHIATRIC TREATMENT

*Wilfrid Llewelyn Jones*

MB BS FRCPych DPM

*Consultant Psychiatrist Emeritus*
*Mapperley Hospital*
*Nottingham*

**William Heinemann Medical Books Ltd**
London

First published 1983
by William Heinemann Medical Books Ltd
23 Bedford Square, London WC1B 3HH

ISBN 0-433-17550-8

*Typeset by Inforum Ltd, Portsmouth*
*Printed in Great Britain by*
*Redwood Burn Ltd, Trowbridge*

# Contents

# *Preface*

I have long been aware of my good fortune in starting on the practice of psychiatry in the early 1940s when the biological treatments introduced ten years earlier were beginning to show their usefulness and to be more widely accepted. These treatments ushered in a new period of advance in psychiatry and were followed by the re-discovery of the better methods of patient management and the organisation of care outside the mental hospitals. The upgrading of standards when the National Health Service was established was a welcome reinforcement. The value of this experience was empha-sised to me when I became engaged in an account of the history of this hospital up to its centenary in 1980. The interest expressed by my younger colleagues in all disciplines suggested to me that their work could become more meaningful to them if they could be made aware of the historical background to the treatments and techniques in which they were engaged. I hope, therefore, that this book will be read not only by psychiatrists in training and their seniors but also by our collaborators and indispensable helpers – general practitioners, psychiatric nurses, occupational therapists, social workers, clinical psychologists and even by some of our patients and their friends. Because of this aim, I hope also that my psychiatric colleagues will forgive the occasional elementary explanations inserted for the general reader and that the same reader will not be discouraged by the references to the medical literature.

All historians of psychiatry in this country are greatly indebted to the late Dr Alexander Walk, Librarian Emeritus of the Royal College of Psychiatrists. I am most grateful to him for his suggestions and for his correction of some of my misapprehensions. I also owe a debt for unfailing help to the librarians of Mapperley Hospital, Brian Spencer and Barbara Astill. Stephen Best of the Central Library, Notting-ham, is a local historian who has readily furnished interesting infor-mation.

Those who have undertaken a work of this kind will know the immeasurable value of a willing and efficient secretary: without the labour of Dorothy Evans this book would never have reached the publisher.

*Mapperley Hospital*                                                   W. L. JONES
*Nottingham*

# Acknowledgements

The following illustrations are reproduced from *Medicine and the Artist (Ars Medica)* by permission of the Philadelphia Museum of Art:

The Physician curing Fantasy
St. Lukes Hospital

Shock treatment by sudden immersion
Magnetic Dispensary
Charcot lecturing on hysteria

are reproduced by courtesty of the Wellcome Trustees.

The portraits of Egas Moniz and I. P. Pavlov and the plate from Esquirol were kindly supplied by the Librarian of The Royal College of Psychiatrists.

The reproduction of Goya's 'El Corral de los Locos' is by courtesy of The Meadows Museum, Southern Methodist University, Dallas, Texas.

The portraits of William Tuke and the Jepsons were supplied by courtesy of The Retreat, York.

The picture of the Freud group is from the Mary Evans Picture Library.

The J. P. Lippincott Company of Philadelphia gave permission for the picture of the mural depicting 'Pinel liberating the Insane'.

The portrait of Dorothea Dix was previously published in *A History of Nursing* by G. Sellewe and C. J. Niresse, London: Kimpton, 1946.

The cover picture is from a seventeenth century Dutch print of a quack treating mental illness. The inscription reads 'Come, come with great rejoicing: here the stones can be cut out of your wife'

# CHAPTER 1

# *Introduction*

Mental illness has been a subject of fear and fascination from time immemorial. That Man's thoughts, feelings and actions should be determined by seemingly irrational and uncontrollable forces has led to a variety of explanations and of reactions to the phenomenon. Theories of causation have been legion: theological and demonological visitations, the influence of heavenly bodies, atmospheric changes, the result of occult forces, the effects of sin and self-indulgence, bodily derangements and even the assent to certain political or economic doctrines.

From ancient to modern times, three aspects of the subject can be discerned when causal theories are examined. The first of these is the immaterial component of the person: soul, spirit, mind, vital element. The second is the physical or bodily component; and third is the effect of the environment or the person's interaction with people, or with nature or with external influences. Contemporary theory has, therefore, always been a major influence on the treatment of mental illness and has made it to a certain extent dependent on the beliefs, sophistication, knowledge and experience of those dealing with it, whether they were priests, doctors, nurses or their erstwhile local equivalents.

Treatment includes the general arrangements for the management and care of patients, and the attitude to this and the amount of concern devoted to it have depended on the social climate of the place and time. Therefore, when we are considering psychiatric treatment, whether it be of an individual or of a whole class of patients, there are psychological, physical, environmental and social factors to take into account. The relative importance of the different factors will vary from case to case. When viewing the history of psychiatric treatment, these factors will have different weights in different places and at different stages of human progress. King Henry VI is represented as a mild, unassertive person, unable to cope with the stresses of the Wars of the Roses, and the treatment of his mental illness was to be shut up in the Tower. Compare him with King George III, a robust character whose mental illness is now thought to have been due to a metabolic defect, porphyria.[1] At first he was put in the care of doctors who subjected him to the bleedings and purgings thought to be effective in those days. Two patients of equal social status: in one the psychological element was most important; in the other it was the physical. Both were treated according to the knowledge and custom of their time. Consider further George III's contemporary, Mary Lamb. Her mental illness was treated by placing her in the loving care of her brother Charles. Part of her treatment was in helping him compile his *Tales from Shakespeare*: he did the tragedies, she did the comedies. The commoner was luckier than the kings. Social factors played only a minor part in determining her treatment.

These are three examples of different approaches to psychiatric treatment: manipulation of the environment, institutional treatment, physical methods and moral treatment which included what we know as psychotherapy and occupational therapy.

### Reference

1. Macalpine I. and Hunter R. (1969). *George III and the Mad-Business* London: Allen Lane.

# I: Somatic Treatments

## CHAPTER 2

# *The Early Physical Treatments*

### Sleep treatment

Sleep, Shakespeare's 'balm of hurt minds', is one of the oldest treatments.

Imhotep (He who comes in peace) was vizier to the Pharaoh about 2900 BC. He is credited with being the architect of the Step Pyramid of Sakkara, but his name is chiefly connected with incubation sleep or temple sleep. Having washed and purified himself, the sick person slept overnight in the temple. After that the priest-physicians would perform religious rituals and interpret the patient's dreams. Imhotep was later deified and temples of his cult were built at Memphis, Thebes and Philae.

Temple sleep was also prominent in the medicine of Ancient Greece. There, the temples honoured Asclepios, the god of healing, who had learned his art from Apollo through Chiron, the patron of surgery. Famous temples of healing were at Cos, Athens and Pergamos; the most famous was at Epidaurus. The snakes in the temples were supposed to lick the eyelids of the sleepers and induce healing dreams.[1] Hence, the symbol of Asclepios was the serpent entwined round his staff. Although mystical and supernatural methods were prominent, the priestly interpretations of dreams could induce confession and relief of conflicts, an effective psychotherapy. In addition, physical treatments in the form of diet, bathing and exercise promoted health.

From the Greeks, the Romans adopted the same methods and there was an Asclepion on the Insula Tiberina in Rome from the third century BC. The legend is that the Romans sent to Epidaurus for help in combatting a plague. As the emissary's ship returned to Rome, a sacred snake from the Greek Temple slipped ashore to the island. The plague died out and the Romans erected a temple to Aesculapius in gratitude.[2] In Roman Britain there was a healing temple at Lydney on the banks of the Severn.

In the early Christian era, incubation persisted, especially round the eastern Mediterranean, and sick persons would spend the night in church. Although McLeod had used bromide sleep for opium addicts in 1908, prolonged sleep or continuous narcosis did not become accepted until after the introduction of the barbiturates. In 1922, Kläsi induced sleep narcosis with somnifaine (di-allyl-barbituric acid) by injection and the treatment would be kept up for seven to ten days. Lightening of the sleep at intervals allowed for toiletting of the patient. Even with the highest standards of nursing care, the risks of pneumonia or suffocation or irreversible coma were not negligible. Another method was the rectal administration, at intervals of three to six hours, of Cloetta's mixture, which was made up of paraldehyde, amylene hydrate, chloral hydrate, alcohol, iso-propylallylbarbituric acid, digitalin and ephedrine hydrochloride.

Kläsi emphasised the importance of following up the narcosis with psychotherapy as the patient was then in a more receptive state. Results were better in anxiety states and mania than in depression and schizophrenia.

Narcosis was used in the Spanish Civil War for the cases of battle exhaustion and neurosis — hyoscine and scopolamine being the drugs of choice. This experience was drawn on in 1940 to treat psychiatric casualties after the evacuation from Dunkirk. Sodium amylobarbitone and paraldehyde were found to be a very effective combination. When chlorpromazine was introduced into pyschiatry its potentiating effect allowed lower and safer doses of barbiturates to be used.

'Electric sleep' and general anaesthesia were produced by high-frequency currents by Leduc in 1902, and narcosis with a current of low amperage has also been used in Russia to treat neuroses. The so-called electronarcosis used in the early 1950s was a variant of electroconvulsive therapy (ECT). It was not without complications and the results were poor.

In contrast to all this is sleep deprivation. Benjamin Rush (1745 – 1813), who is regarded as the father of American psychiatry, used to keep disturbed patients standing awake for 24 hours. As a treatment for depression, sleep deprivation has a more recent history. Electro-encephalographic (EEG) recordings show that there are two qualitatively different kinds of sleep: these are non-rapid eye movement (NREM) or orthodox sleep, and paradoxical sleep which is accompanied by rapid eye movements (REM). They alternate throughout the night in normal individuals. A study by Vogel (1975) showed that patients deprived of REM sleep, as observed in a sleep laboratory with continuous EEG recording, were relieved of depressive symptoms and their activity improved.[3,4]

## Hydrotherapy

Water, one of the four elements, has always had a fascination for healers. Its cleansing action has particularly appealed to those holding the view that mental illness is the result of sin, uncleanness or impurity. Water could be used either actually or symbolically to wash away the offence. Thus, washing and purification were an essential preliminary to the healing process. The inscription over the entrance to the temple at Epidaurus read 'Pure must he be who enters the fragrant temple; purity means to think nothing but holy thoughts'.

In those places where there was a spring, and temples and hospitals tended to be built next to a source of fresh water, the mineral content of the water could produce purgation or promote inner cleanliness. Bathing and the taking of the waters were therefore important in temple healing. In later centuries, spas were set up and the waters of Bad Oeyenhausen, Schlangenbad and Church Stretton have been recommended for nervous diseases.

In the eighteenth century in Finland, a bath at the iron spa at Kupitaa was tried before a patient was sent to the Seili Mental Hospital.[5] In modern times the bathing of the sick at Lourdes is an important adjunct to the spiritual exercises.

Perfumed and medicated baths were prescribed by Arab physicians in the Middle Ages. The soothing effect of warm water has always been recognised and continuous baths for excited or agitated patients were long in vogue. It was recognised that in some cases restraint and observation were necessary: restraint to prevent the melancholic patient attempting suicide by drowning, and observation for signs of circulatory collapse. The heat was also commended for opening the pores and getting rid of toxins through the skin. Dr

Sheppard's Turkish Bath Treatment at Friern Hospital in the nineteenth century was highly thought of and copied, and was only discontinued in the First World War because of the expense of the heating.[6] The cold douche and the wet pack were used for the overactive patient. The latter was as much a method of restraint as an application of healing fluid. The cold douche had a shock effect as well as a calming effect.

Jean Baptiste van Helmont (1577–1644), following the old doctrine of the antagonism between water and hydrophobia which is insanity, recommended suspending the patient head first in water until unconscious and then reviving him. Thomas Willis (1621–75), physician of Oxford and London, directed that a 'furious maid' 'should be drenched into the depth of the River'. Hermann Boerhaave (1668–1738) was Professor of Medicine at Leyden. He wrote '. . . if melancholia go so far that the agitation of the cerebral fluid causes the patient to go raving mad, it is called mania'. He went on: 'Plunging into the sea, immersion for as long as it can be borne, is the chief remedy'. A report in the *Journal of Mental Science* for 1880 indicates that their words were heeded even much later. A manic woman of Killarney was bound and towed behind a rowing boat. She developed pneumonia, recovered from that and from the mania.

In the 1930s, after the Mental Treatment Act 1930 permitted the admission of voluntary patients to mental hospitals, some hospitals built new separate admission units for such patients and elaborate hydrotherapy departments were a feature of these. It would be interesting to know if the sauna, with its combination of moist heat, cold shock and skin stimulation, has ever been used in pyschiatric treatment. It has had its place in the treatment of allergies in Finland.

## Bloodletting and blood transfusion

Blood figures in myths, folklore and religious belief all over the world: blood is life and, according to Rabelais, 'Life consisteth in blood'.

Empedocles (504 – 443 BC) held that everything was composed in varying degree of the four elements — earth, fire, air, water — whose qualities were cold, heat, dryness and moisture. After this doctrine of the four elements there developed the theory of the four humours in the body. These humours were found in blood which, when shed, showed a bright red surface layer (blood the humour), then the

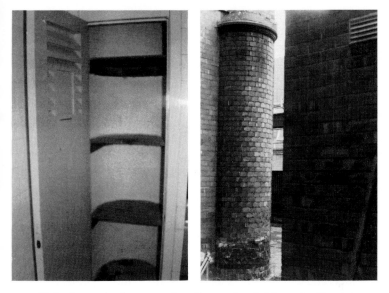

*Hydrotherapy douche converted to a linen cupboard; Mapperley Hospital, Nottingham*

separated light yellow serum (yellow bile), then the dark jelly of red cells in fibrin (black bile), and then the buffy coat of white blood cells and platelets (phlegm). Each humour was formed and stored in a different part of the body: the blood in the heart, the yellow bile in the liver, the black bile in the spleen, and the phlegm in the brain.

Excess of phlegm was blamed for most diseases but melancholy was ascribed to an excess of black bile. Therefore, drawing off whole blood would remove the offending humour. Thus bloodletting became a well-entrenched treatment from the Hippocratic era to the early nineteenth century. In the Middle Ages, two theories of blood-letting were in opposition. The derivative method of Hippocrates was to take blood from a vein near the diseased part and on the same side of the body. The Arabic revulsion method was to take blood from a vein at a distance from the diseased part and on the opposite side of the body.[7] After William Harvey published his book *De Motu Cordis* in 1628, establishing the circulation of the blood, bloodletting was even more enthusiastically practised. Guy Patin, Professor of Medicine at Paris and an opponent of Harvey, quoted approvingly in one of his Letters the words of the lyric poet Joachim du Bellay 'Oh good, oh holy, oh divine bloodletting'.[8]

In the eighteenth century, Theophile Bonet bled a manic girl 30 times in ten days. Not surprisingly, she died, but apparently Bonet learnt nothing from this or from the autopsy. Two kings of England, Charles II and George III suffered at the hands of dedicated phlebotomists.

Marshall Hall, a successful physician and pioneer neurologist of the nineteenth century, denounced bloodletting and described the lancet as 'minute instrument of mighty mischief', whereas Bryan Crowther in his *Practical Remarks on Insanity* (1811) called it 'a very communicative sort of instrument' because it tended to invalidate the claim of phrenitis to be considered to be the general cause of mania: its existence would be indicated by the appearance of the blood drawn from the patient. In a footnote, he says: 'The curable patients in Bethlem Hospital are regularly bled about the commencement of June, and the latter end of July'. This is explained by his quotation from *Burdin's Medical Studies*: 'Warm seasons have a striking influence upon the return of the paroxysm in mania'. In another passage 'the exploded theory of revulsion' is referred to.

There were two other methods of bloodletting. Leeches (the bloodsucking variety is *Hirudo sanguisuga*) would be applied to the part of the body chosen as most appropriate. Leeches round the anus were prescribed for melancholia according to 'the exploded theory of revulsion'. Arabs were forbidden to apply leeches to the nape of the neck: this would produce loss of memory by action on the posterior part of the brain, according to the Koran.

The other method was cupping. In dry cupping a glass cup, warmed, would be applied closely to the shaven head or afflicted area. As the air in the cup cooled and contracted, blood was drawn to the skin and away from the internal parts where it was presumed there was congestion. In wet cupping, the skin under the cup was scarified to allow escape of excess blood.

In contrast to all this, blood transfusion as a cure for mental illness was first attempted by Richard Lower (1631–91) in 1667.[9] Samuel Pepys, as a Fellow of the Royal Society, describes the patient as 'a little frantic'. When he saw him afterwards, although the patient claimed to be a new man, he wrote 'but he is cracked a little in his head'. Sir George Ent (1604–1689), a friend and legatee of William Harvey, had proposed that a patient from Bethlem be selected for the experiment, but Dr Thomas Allen, the physician there, refused the Society's request. In the same year Jean Baptiste Denis, physician to Louis XIV, treated a patient in Paris by drawing off blood and then running in calf's blood on two successive days. The subsequent cure was said to be confirmed by all the professors of the Ecole de Chirurgie.[10] That patient was luckier than Denis' patient of the year before who, previously weakened by a massive bloodletting, died after a transfusion of lamb's blood. It was thought, following Aristotle, that new blood would make a new man. The practice continued during the next two centuries, vying with bloodletting. Not until Landsteiner demonstrated the blood groups in 1900 were the failures explained as being due to the incompatability of the transfused red blood cells with the patient's own.

## Shock treatment

When mental illness was considered to be the result of demoniacal possession, shock treatments to expel the evil spirit were popular. Flogging, purgation and induced vomiting were the usual methods. The methods of purgation and emesis were the same when the rationale was to get rid of morbid humours or toxins.

The exasperated relative who has failed by argument to change the mind of the deluded patient says 'Oh, I could shake him!' Another will beseech the patient 'Why don't you snap out of it?' These are examples of the thought that a sharp sudden shock will somehow rearrange the disordered mental mechanism into order again. Even Pinel, who unfettered the patients in the Bicêtre, believed in the efficacy of a sudden fright; and Conolly, the advocate of non-restraint, included the cold douche in his treatments. Suddenly surprising the patient with a plunge into cold water was practised in several eras from ancient times to the nineteenth century. Boats were constructed which would break up and force patients to swim to the shore in the cold water and there were bridges which would collapse when patients were crossing them. The 'douche ascendante' at the Salpêtrière was a stream of cold water directed on the anus of the naked, seated, unsuspecting patient.

A patient could be subjected to more prolonged stress by forcible rotation which could produce dizziness, nausea, vomiting, bowel evacuation and even unconsciousness. It may have been the ecstasies and states of altered consciousness attained by whirling dervishes

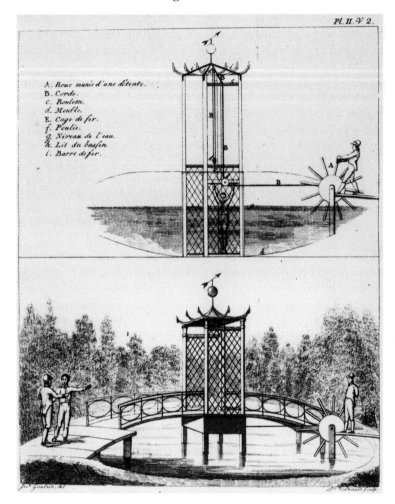

*Shock treatment by sudden immersion. From Joseph Guislain:* Traité sur
l'aliénation mentale, *vol 2, 1826*

which gave Avicenna, the great Islamic physician of the tenth century, the idea of a rotating chair. The same thing was used by
Benjamin Rush and an elaborate rotary machine is illustrated in
Joseph Guislain's *Traité sur l'aliénation mentale et sur les hospices des
aliénés* of 1826. Celsus, the Roman physician, recommended swing-
ing the patient and frightening the patient. Erasmus Darwin

(1731–1802) recommended putting the patient on a rotating disc with his head towards the centre or towards the periphery, according to the supposed cause. Congestion in the brain was relieved with the head at the outer edge. For congestion in internal organs, the patient lay with his feet outward.

In more modern times shock treatment consisted of putting the patient under stress, the idea being that the autonomic nervous system was thereby mobilised to restore equilibrium. In the 1930s, Gellhorn used a carbon dioxide and oxygen mixture and Himwich used inhalations of nitrogen to produce a temporary anoxia in schizophrenic patients. The carbon dioxide treatment was revived by Meduna in 1950 for the treatment of neurosis. Injections of acetylcholine were calculated to reduce overactivity of the sympathetic division of the autonomic system in anxiety states, a treatment tried by Minsch and revived by Lopez-Ibor in 1950. The shock effect was to stop the heart beat momentarily. The results were not very encouraging and the treatment did not flourish long.

## Electrical treatment

The derivation of the word electric from the Greek word for amber, reminds us that Thales of Alexandria (c. 600 BC) discovered that amber, when rubbed, attracted certain other substances. The electric torpedo or cramp fish was known to the Greeks and Romans for its stupefying and blunting effects and Galen prepared 'an oil from the dead animal', according to Sir John Pringle in 1774.[11]

William Gilbert (1544–1603), who was physician to Queen Elizabeth I, wrote a treatise on magnetism, and in the following century electric friction machines and condensers and the Leyden jar were devised.

In the eighteenth century, electric machines were used in medicine. John Wesley (1703–1791), who was concerned with the physical as well as the spiritual health of his flocks, records that he bought one such machine in 1756 and that it brought immediate help for several disorders. Then he went on to wonder why physicians did not consider how far bodily disorders were caused or influenced by the mind. Editions of his *Primitive Physick* after 1760 contained a section on electric treatment.

Towards the end of the eighteenth century, electrical treatment became available, and research into its use was carried out. The

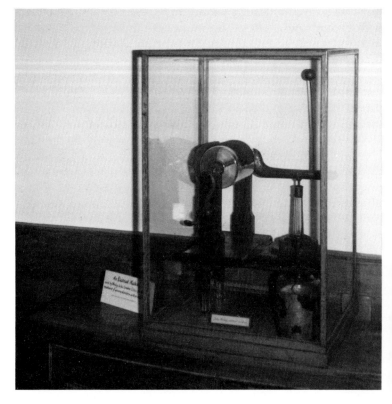

*John Wesley's Electrical Machine*

Electrical Dispensary in London was founded in 1793. At Notting-ham General Hospital, electrical treatment was available on payment of sixpence. John Birch (1745–1815), surgeon to St Thomas' Hospital, London, reported in 1792 the cure of two cases of melancholy by application of electricity to the head. Benjamin Franklin (1706–1790), an early experimenter with electricity, accidentally knocked himself out twice and then suggested 'trying the practice on mad people'.

Luigi Galvani (1737–98), Professor of Anatomy at Bologna, pub-lished his experiments on the electric stimulation of frogs' muscles in 1791. In 1804, his nephew Aldini claimed to have cured two cases of melancholia by the application of electricity. At the mental hospital of Aversa, near Naples, which was founded in 1813, electrotherapy was used for several years[12] and later it was used in Poland, Tasmania and at the Salpêtrière in Paris.

A.H. Newth, writing in the *Journal of Mental Science* in 1885, described the continuous current as sedative and the intermittent current as stimulating. One electrode was placed on the head, the other over the cervical spine: they were not both to be placed on the head.

Other applications of electricity in the early decades of the twentieth century were diathermy and ultraviolet light. The latter was being used in the treatment of tuberculosis and cases of this infection were not uncommon in mental hospitals. Its use extended to be a general tonic for the debilitated patient and it was still being prescribed in mental hospitals in Britain in the 1940s.

In the 1930s diathermy was being applied to restless patients, the soothing effect being equated with that of the warm bath.

Following the introduction of electric convulsive therapy, various methods of electrostimulatory non-convulsive treatment were tried. Because of the unpleasant nature of the faradic currents used, the patients had to be treated under short-acting barbiturate narcosis, and it was concluded that any favourable results were due to that rather than to the electricity.

A paper in the *British Journal of Psychiatry* in 1974 on the effects of small electric currents on depressive symptoms showed that any improvement was temporary.

# References

1. Guthrie D. (1945). *A History of Medicine*. London: Nelson.
2. Risley M. (1962). *The House of Healing*. London: Robert Hale.
3. Vogel G.W. (1975). A Review of REM sleep deprivation *Archives of General Psychiatry*; **32**:749.
4. British Medical Journal (1975). Depression and curtailment of sleep (leading article). *British Medical Journal*; **4**:543.
5. Acte K. (1945). Use of water as a mode of psychiatric treatment. Quoted in *Psychiatric Briefs* (1977) vol. 10 No. 1. Welwyn Garden City: Smith Kline and French Laboratories.
6. Hunter R.A. and Macalpine I. (1974). *Psychiatry for the Poor*. London: Dawson.
7. Richardson R.G. (1975) *Blood — A very special juice*. Queenborough: Abbott Laboratories.
8. Zilboorg G. (1941). *A History of Medical Psychology*. New York: W.W. Norton.

9. Hunter R.A., Macalpine I. (1963). In *Three Hundred Years of Psychiatry 1535—1860,* p. 154. London: Oxford University Press.
10. Keynes G. (1967). Tercentenary of blood transfusion. *British Medical Journal*; 4:410.
11. Hunter R.A. Macalpine I. (1963). *Op cit.,* p. 534.
12. Mora G. (1975). In *World History of Psychiatry* (Howells J.G., ed.) p. 66. London: Baillière Tindall.

# CHAPTER 3

# *Epilepsy and its Treatment*

The word epilepsy is derived from the Greek, meaning 'to take hold of', hence the use of the word seizure to describe its main manifestation.

Lacking our present knowledge, preceding generations found epilepsy mysterious, awe-inspiring and fearful, especially as seizures range from petit mal, with its momentary periods of blankness, through the terrifying convulsions of grand mal, to the sometimes prolonged periods of confusion, disordered behaviour and altered consciousness of psychomotor epilepsy. Allied to these are the irresistible sleep tendency in narcolepsy and the brief attacks of paralysis in cataplexy. The suddenness and unpredictability of seizures have added to the mystery and fear. From antiquity to the relatively recent past, these phenomena were seen as divine retribution for wickedness or due to possession by spirits or devils or to the influence of the moon. The Greeks called epilepsy 'the sacred disease'. Hippocrates (460–355 BC), whose medical teaching was based on observation and logical reasoning, wrote of epilepsy 'It is not in my opinion any more divine or more sacred than other diseases, but has a natural cause, and its supposed divine origin is due to man's experience . . .'. Although he attributed it to a malfunction of the brain due to an excess of phlegm (one of the four humours), the impossibility of verifying this did not allow the rational explanation to prevail against the magical.

John of Gaddesden (1280–1361), thought to be the original of Chaucer's *Doctor of Physick*, was said to conquer epilepsy with a necklace. John of Arderne (1307–1390), who had been an army surgeon at the Battle of Crecy, used a charm: 'the words Melchior,

Jasper and Balthazar to be written in blood from the little finger of the patient' and the paper worn for a month, and the patient was to say daily three Paternosters and three Aves.

At Wrexham, there was a well where epileptic sufferers washed and threw in fourpence. After walking thrice round the well and thrice round the church reciting Paternosters, they spent the night in church with a Bible for a pillow.

Other ancient remedies, such as hippopotamus testicles and tortoise blood, gave way to purges and enemas and fomentations calculated to drive out the possessing demons, a theory conveniently backed up by the Biblical story of the Gadarene Swine.

Jean Riolan, Professor of Anatomy in Paris and an opponent of William Harvey's views on the circulation, wrote in 1610 'It is not necessary for us to have recourse to a demon as the last refuge of ignorance since we have a natural cause'. The enlightenment of the eighteenth century did not end the myths attached to epilepsy. Masturbation and sexual excess were regarded as the commonest causes of fits, and castration was advised.

In 1857, Sir Charles Locock reported that because of the association of fits with hysteria and the menses he had given potassium bromide and it had been effective in 14 out of 15 cases.[1] Its effectiveness as an anticonvulsant was then gradually realised. The next advance was in 1912 when Hauptmann showed the value of phenobarbitone.

Mental changes, either the development of a sly, unctuous, prolix, malicious personality or a frank psychosis, develop in some epileptic patients. There has been a controversy as to whether these changes were due to the effects of frequent seizures, resulting in defective circulation in the brain and reduction of oxygen supply to the nerve cells, or to an underlying general disturbance of brain function of which both the fits and the mental changes were symptoms. In the nineteenth century and the first half of the twentieth despite the use of bromide and phenobarbitone, most mental hospitals had a ward of disturbed epileptics.

Consideration of changes in blood chemistry which inhibited seizures and of the structure of phenobarbitone led Merritt and Putnam to screen a series of phenyl compounds. They found one, diphenylhydantoin, which was non-toxic, non-hypnotic and anti-convulsant. They reported their original results to the meeting of the American Medical Association at San Francisco in 1938.[2] The news quickly spread and as early as July 1939 there were favourable reports to the Annual Meeting of the Royal Medico-Psychological Association in London. The better control of seizures has resulted in the virtual disappearance of disturbed epileptics from the wards of mental hospitals. Some credit must also be given to better obstetric and perinatal care which has reduced the incidence of birth injury to the brain. The lessened incidence of serious febrile illness in childhood as a result of preventive inoculation and of antibiotic treatment has also contributed.

Surgery has also had its place in the treatment of epilepsy. Sir William Osler (1849–1919), physician and scholar and Regius Professor of Medicine at Oxford, recorded in his *Principles and Practice of Medicine* that some 30 types of operation, not necessarily on the head, have been reported to alleviate seizures.

Archaeological finds from a variety of places and cultures provide evidence of trephining operations in primitive times. Operations on the skull to evacuate evil spirits would be a logical sequence of belief in demoniacal possession.

Brain surgery began towards the end of the nineteenth century. Wilder Penfield, the great Canadian neurosurgeon, has described how he operated in 1927 to remove a scar on the brain and how he then went to collaborate with his illustrious contemporary Otfrid Foerster (1873–1941) in Breslau on the surgical removal of atrophic epileptogenic lesions. The development of the electro-encephalograph by Hans Berger (1873–1941) in 1929 led to better understanding of the electrical activity of the brain in health and in disease and was a help in identifying the position of pathological foci from which epileptic discharges originated.

Between 1928 and 1966, Penfield and his successors performed 1690 operations on 1450 epileptic patients in the Montreal Neurological Institute. Of the first 115 patients between 1929 and 1939, 43% were free or nearly free of fits.[3]

Clinical and EEG observation and the pathological examination of post-mortem material combined to clarify the concept of the complicated attacks with psychiatric features which constitute psychomotor epilepsy. These are now recognised to be due to morbid tissue, frequently, but not exclusively, in the temporal lobe of the brain. Surgical excision of the diseased areas has produced relief for patients whose symptoms have not been controlled by medication. Some cases of infantile hemiplegia due to birth injury, with unrelieved fits, have been improved by removal of the whole of the cerebral cortex on the affected side. The loss of a grossly disturbed area has reduced seizures, reduced the interference of the malfunctioning cortex with healthier parts of the brain and has not made worse the partial paralysis.

## References

1. Locock C. (1857). Fifty two cases of epilepsy observed by the author. *Lancet*; **i**:529.
2. Merritt H.H. and Putnam T.J. (1958). Sodium phenylhydantoinate in the treatment of convulsive disorders. *Journal of the American Medical Association*; **11**:1068.
3. Penfield W. (1958). Pitfalls and success in the surgical treatment of focal epilepsy. *British Medical Journal*; **1**:669.

# CHAPTER 4

# The Later Physical Treatments

## Fever therapy

Fever therapy is another form of shock treatment. It was frequently noted that the symptoms of a mental illness would remit while the patient was in the grip of a fever. In the seventeenth century, Thomas Willis saw that a fever cured a man of stupidity and, in the eighteenth century, the insane in England were sent to the Fens to contract malaria for its beneficial results.[1] Means of raising the patient's temperature were sought. Sterile abscesses were induced by the subcutaneous injection of irritants such as turpentine. In Hungary in 1909, Gyula Donath suggested sodium nucleicum; in Denmark in 1924, sulfosin (sulphur in oil) was used; a report of the Commissioners of the Board of Control in 1934 mentions injections of pyrifer, which was a bacterial vaccine developed in Germany, and sterile milk. One to three series of eight to ten injections were recommended. The treatment was chiefly used in schizophrenia.[2] However, the most successful fever treatment was the induction of malaria in the treatment of general paralysis of the insane (GPI), or dementia paralytica, a psychosis identified as a syphilitic infection of the brain when the Wasserman test was introduced in 1907, although the presence of spirochaetes in the brain was not demonstrated until 1913. Illustrious neuroluetics, to borrow Dr Macdonald Critchley's phrase,[3] include Jules de Goncourt, Guy de Maupassant, Dan Leno and General Gamelin.[4] Paul Ehrlich (1854–1915) introduced salvarsan or 606 (it was the 606th compound tested in his quest for 'the magic bullet') in 1909. It was effective against the primary and secondary stages of syphilitic infection but could not pass from the blood into the brain tissue. Julius Wagner-Jauregg (1857–1940) in Vienna had been interested in the problem of GPI which, untreated, led to dementia, debilitation and death, from 1887. In 1917 he had admitted to his ward a soldier suffering from malaria and he took the opportunity of inoculating some GPI patients with malarial blood. In benign tertian malaria, the appearance of successive waves of parasites in the blood produces a febrile reaction every second day. The results were encouraging in that the progress of the GPI was halted. By the end of the First World War, his experience enabled him to standardise the treatment at eight febrile attacks before aborting the malarial infection.

The treatment was first given in this country at Whittingham Mental Hospital, Lancashire, in 1922 with the help of the Professor of Tropical Medicine at Liverpool, and later other hospitals took it up.[5] In his Presidential Address to the Royal Medico-Psychological Association in 1956, Dr T.P. Rees recalled that he spent his first four years in psychiatry in a mental hospital where malaria treatment was not allowed because the medical superintendent feared that the mosquitoes in the local pond might become infected! At Horton Hospital, Epsom, the London County Council established a clinic for the treatment of patients from all its mental hospitals. At this hospital there was also a research laboratory, directed by P.G. Shute, who progressed from baker's lad to internationally known scientist. From there, other hospitals could obtain infected mosquitoes. It was, however, also the practice to convey the malaria from patient to patient by injections of blood obtained at the height of a paroxysm. Neighbouring hospitals would collaborate. A 1927 entry in the Superintendent's Journal of Mapperley Hospital, Nottingham, records 'Today Dr Alexander regained our original strain of malarial blood from Leicester City Mental Hospital'. The strain had been obtained on 29th December 1925 when a patient was sent to Wadsley Mental Hospital, Sheffield, for inoculation.

In the late 1930s, the Kettering Hypertherm was another method of inducing fever. It was built at the Kettering Institute in Dayton, Ohio. Patients were placed in a chamber with hot air circulating through it and kept at a temperature of 41°C for eight hours.

Before the end of the 1939–45 War, penicillin was being used successfully to treat all stages of syphilis and it was not long before fever therapy was shown to be unnecessary.

## Insulin treatment

The isolation of insulin by Banting and Best in 1922 gave, of course, new life to sufferers from diabetes mellitus. It also put into the hands of the pyschiatrists a substance which could powerfully alter the body metabolism, thereby giving the hope of attacking by physical means some of the hitherto insoluble problems of mental illness. Broadly speaking, the action of insulin is to enable the cells of the body to use carbohydrate (glucose) which is absorbed from food or released from the liver and which is circulating in the blood. An excess of insulin may come from an injection into a healthy person or as an overdose in a diabetic or from overactivity of the insulin-producing cells of the pancreas. The effect is to reduce the amount of glucose in the blood and therefore the amount available to the body cells, particularly the brain cells. This condition of hypoglycaemia starts with faintness, sweating and tremors and can proceed, depending on the dose of insulin, to drowsiness, mental confusion, sopor or sleep and even as far as coma and death. These symptoms can be reversed by the swift provision of glucose to raise the blood sugar level. Thus a small dose can stimulate the autonomic nervous system, more will produce sedation and a still larger dose loss of consciousness.

In 1923, it was noted that depressions cleared up in some insulin-treated diabetics. Then insulin with glucose was used to improve the nutrition of debilitated patients. There were reports of the use of hypoglycaemia to relieve the symptoms of delirium tremens, and in 1928 Manfred Sakel (1900–1957) was one of those who used it to mitigate withdrawal symptoms in morphine addicts. At this time, hypoglycaemic sopor or coma was a complication to be warned against. However, Sakel thought that he could use the parasympathetic overactivity in morphine withdrawal. Animal experiments convinced him that insulin shock was not dangerous and that it could be controlled. Encouraging results in the treatment of excited patients, including schizophrenics, convinced him that he had made an important discovery. His theory was that the illness was due to abnormal cell connections in the brain. The hypoglycaemic shocks, by repetition, interrupted these connections and allowed the innate tendency to homeostasis (that is, the steady state) to be re-established. This was following the ancient doctrine of *vis medicatrix naturae*.

In 1933, Sakel returned to Vienna from Berlin and worked as an unpaid assistant to the University Department of Psychiatry. He and Hans Hoff (later Professor) successfully treated a private patient of Professor Wagner-Jauregg with insulin, and then a second patient. This enabled them to interest Professor Otto Potzl, the Professor of Psychiatry, in the treatment and he gave them facilities to develop the coma method and supported them in the face of the criticism engendered by the publication of their results.[6]

In 1936, favourable reports on two large series of patients were published in Vienna and in Switzerland and the treatment was in use in three American hospitals. In the same year a commissioner of the Board of Control, Dr Isobel Wilson, went to Vienna and returned with a satisfactory report of her findings to psychiatrists in Britain.[7]

Examination of the results of the treatment established that the best responses were obtained in schizophrenic patients who had a history of less than two years of illness, whose illness had had an acute rather than an insidious onset, who had positive symptoms of disturbed behaviour and delusions and hallucinations rather than negative symptoms of apathy and anergia. Treatment was best given in a specialised unit to a small group of patients by experienced medical and nursing staff. This ensured the maintenance of enthusiasm and high standards of care. The insulin treatment had to be supplemented by the other usual forms of psychiatric care — the consideration of psychological factors, explanation, reassurance, occupation and social rehabilitation.

In the 1939–45 War, insulin coma treatment suffered because of the reductions in medical and nursing staffs and the lessened availability of insulin and glucose. A solution of glucose was given by stomach tube to terminate the coma. In some clinics it was replaced by a potato purée which provided easily available carbohydrate, although after-shocks (recurrence of low blood sugar) were more common. Sub-coma insulin treatment was used by those who had observed improvements in patients before the coma treatment came in and by those who did not have the facilities for close observation and nursing which the full treatment demanded.

The results in schizophrenia, even when supplemented by convulsion treatment, were not so good. There was, however, a useful place for sub-coma treatment. Patients, service and civilian, who had developed anxiety and tension as a result of severe and protracted stress, were treated. Acute symptoms subsided but depression and neurotic personality features were not improved. Drs William Sargant and Eliot Slater reported their good results in 1940 and incorporated their experience in their book *An Introduction to Physical Methods of Treatment in Psychiatry*.

The sedative effect of the insulin, and the stimulation of appetite and the regaining of lost weight improved the patient's general condition and rendered him more responsive to psychotherapeutic measures. The enhancement of body bulk had been a feature of the Weir Mitchell treatment in the later decades of the nineteenth century.

After 1945, insulin coma treatment picked up again. It was severely criticised in a 1953 paper in the *Lancet* entitled 'The Insulin Myth' in which the good results were ascribed to the strong suggestive effect of the technique together with the enthusiasm of a dedicated staff, the inculcation of a group morale in a special unit and the 'total push' adjuvant treatment.[8] The idea of an 'elite' was expressed by a patient in an American hospital.

> This is the psycho
> The home of the buzz and the prod
> Where electric shock patients
> Speak only to insulins
> The insulins only to God.

Another paper in 1957 demonstrated equal results from insulin coma and barbiturate narcosis.[9] The treatment declined after that. The reasons for the decline were the poor selection of patients, neglect of technique, and the scamping of rehabilitation.

The most important factor in the decline was the introduction of the neuroleptics, the major tranquillisers which controlled the symptoms of schizophrenia and were easier and safer to administer. They, like insulin coma, put the patient into a state where re-educative and re-socialising methods of rehabilitation could have an effect.

## Convulsion treatment

Several strands can be discerned in the reasoning that epileptic convulsions can be theraputic. It was noted when epilepsy was poorly controlled that a period of mental disturbance sometimes preceded a seizure and that it subsided after a seizure. A temporary improvement was noted in some psychotic patients after a seizure. Some of these, in the 1920s, would be patients who had been treated with heavy doses of barbiturates which had been too quickly withdrawn and who thereby suffered a barbiturate withdrawal seizure.

One story is that the unsuccessful treatment of epilepsy with the serum of schizophrenics by Nyiro, a Hungarian psychiatrist, suggested the reverse: the treatment of schizophrenia with epilepsy! Certainly there was the idea that epilepsy and schizophrenia were biologically incompatible.[10] Glaus in 1931 reported that the incidence of epilepsy in schizophrenic patients, 1.3 per 1000, was lower than in the general population.

Ladislas Meduna in Budapest treated patients with intramuscular injections of camphor in oil. Nausea and vomiting were frequent complications and the impossibility of forecasting the time or the length of the convulsions led to his abandoning this method. Then he used a soluble synthetic camphor preparation known in Europe as Cardiazol (Metrazol in the USA). It was injected directly into the bloodstream. Its drawbacks were that it could be painful and cause thrombosis of the vein used. In spite of rapid injection, there was an interval between the injection and the onset of the convulsion. During this interval the patient could experience great anxiety and a feeling of impending death. In the convulsion the patient was unconscious and therefore had no memory of it, but the preceding horror was remembered and it would be prolonged when no convulsion followed. Patients would go to great lengths and claim spurious improvement in order to avoid further treatment. Other drugs such as picrotoxin and triazol were tried in the hope of ameliorating the experience.[11]

The results of convulsion treatment in schizophrenia were encouraging but often the early improvement was not maintained. It became apparent that depressive symptoms were being relieved more than other symptoms. When the treatment was tried in severe melancholia, the results were more impressive and lasting. A patient, who had been severely depressed for nine months and who was one of the first treated with Cardiazol, was so much better after two treatments that he threatened to sue the hospital for negligence in not having got him out of his misery sooner.[12]

### Electroconvulsive therapy

The search for less unpleasant methods of producing a convulsion led to the use of electricity. Ugo Cerletti, engaged in psychiatric research in Rome, was told of Meduna's convulsion treatment by a German-Jewish refugee, Dr Lothar Kalinowsky, and introduced it into his own clinic. He had been studying the changes in the brain cells of animals after convulsions and, to avoid the possible toxic effects of drugs, had been using an electric current to produce convulsions with one electrode in the mouth and another in the rectum. Some animals died of cardiac arrest and trials for safety showed what was the smallest effective dose of electricity and the shortest effective time: 70 volts for 0.1 seconds.

The next step was to produce a generalised convulsion resembling that produced by Cardiazol, and the experiments were done on pigs at the slaughterhouse by applying the electrodes to both sides of the head. Here the object was to find the amount of current needed to produce a fatal outcome, and Cerletti found that there was a big difference between the convulsant dose and the electrocuting dose. He thus decided that it would be safe to try it on a human being.

The first patient to be treated was a chronic schizophrenic who was admitted from the Stazione Termini, the main railway station of Rome, where he had arrived from Northern Italy. He was talking gibberish and could not give any account of himself. He was given the 70-volt shock for one-tenth of a second from a machine devised by Cerletti's assistant, Lucio Bini. The patient had a spasm, did not lose consciousness and burst into song. Cerletti announced that he was going to give a stronger shock and his assistants demurred. The patient said clearly 'Non una seconda. Mortifera.' (Not a second one. It will kill me.). Cerletti took the responsibility and the first electroconvulsive treatment was achieved. This was in November 1937.[13] Bini had announced the possibility of electrically induced convulsion treatment at the first International Conference on the Treatment of Schizophrenia which had met a few months previously at Munsingen in Switzerland.

As the use of convulsion treatment spread, concern was felt when unwanted complications were discovered. Complaints of pain in the back led to the discovery by x-ray of crush fractures of vertebrae. X-rays of non-complaining patients showed that some had fractures which did not give rise to symptoms. An investigation of an epileptic population in 1939 showed that some of them had the same fractures and no disability had been caused. Occasional dislocations and fractures of the humerus also occurred and means were sought of damping down the muscular contractions. Curare, the drug used by the

South American Indians to paralyse their prey when hunting, was first used by Bennett in 1940. The paralysing effect was neutralised after the seizure by the intravenous injection of Prostigmin, but fatalities occurred because of the central effects of the curare in some patients. A refined extract, d-tubocurarine, proved to be safer. Other drugs were developed and used, not only in ECT but also in general anaesthesia in surgery where muscle relaxation was achieved with lower doses of anaesthetic. These were decamethonium iodide, gallamine triethyliodide (Flaxedil), and suxethonium bromide (Brevidil E) and succinylcholine chloride (Scoline). The last two, being of short action and requiring no antidote, are in use today. As the effect of the muscle relaxant is to paralyse not only the muscles of the limbs and trunk, but also the muscles of respiration, the effect on the conscious patient is to produce a feeling of suffocation. For this reason the patient is first put to sleep with a short-acting barbiturate — thiopentone (Pentothal) and, more recently, methohexitone sodium (Brietal) — before the relaxant is injected. Until natural respiration is re-established, breathing is assisted with oxygen under gentle positive pressure.

The relative ease and acceptability of modified ECT led to its widespread use. It revolutionised the treatment of melancholia, an illness in which suicide is always a possibility. No longer were groups of silent, miserable patients to be seen in admission wards. The Suicidal Caution Card, on which each nurse had to sign that he or she knew that the patient needed constant observation 24 hours per day, became a thing of the past and tube-feeding of the resistive self-starving patient was no longer necessary. Electroconvulsive therapy was also found effective in mania. Here the dangers were of exhaustion due to overactivity and dehydration, and toxicity due to the heavy doses of sedatives required. Given once or twice daily on successive days, ECT produced rapid improvement and rendered the patient susceptible to proper nursing care.

There can be too much of a good thing and so it was with ECT. It could produce panic and lifelong horror of the treatment in the mis-diagnosed neurotic patient. A few enthusiasts misused it intensively and desperately in the hope of curing hysteria and chronic schizophrenia. The results were disappointing and in some cases fatal.

Although the newer drugs have lessened the need for ECT, it still has a place in the psychiatric armamentarium. Those outside psychiatry who would ban its use have experienced neither the responsibility of caring for psychiatric patients nor the personal suffering of a depressive illness.

In 1958, a report on hexafluorodiethyl ether (Indoklon) showed that it could be used for convulsive therapy. It is a volatile, non-inflammable liquid. Given by inhalation, a small concentration in the aspired air produces convulsions and larger concentrations produce anaesthesia. Its advantages were that it was less unpleasant than Cardiazol and the patients felt less confused and happier after treatment. The disadvantages were that it could not be used with a relaxant which paralysed respiration and that it produced a second convulsion in about 25% of patients. It did not replace ECT.

## Surgery

A Swiss psychiatrist, Burckhardt, operated on a violent patient in 1888, reasoning that sensory stimuli of abnormal intensity were reaching the motor area in the parietal lobe of the cerebral cortex and causing the behaviour disturbance. Therefore, he severed the connecting fibres between the sensory and motor areas in a series of four operations before the patient became quiet and co-operative. In another operation he interrupted connections between the frontal lobes and central areas and the patient lost his aggressiveness. Three more patients, all of poor prognosis, had temporal lobe excisions to relieve auditory hallucinations, but without benefit.

That Burckhardt was able to plan and carry out such operations was due to the work of pioneers before him. The greatest advances which have occurred in medicine were made in the nineteenth century and they are the prevention of epidemic disease, the discovery of anaesthesia and the control of sepsis. Others, less spectacular but no less important, are the development of physiology, bacteriology and cellular pathology.

Anaesthesia, the name proposed by Oliver Wendell Holmes (1809–1894), was foreshadowed by Sir Humphrey Davy (1778–1829) in 1799 when he suggested that nitrous oxide 'seemed capable of destroying pain' and could be used in surgical operations. Michael Faraday (1791–1867), Davy's assistant at the Royal Institution, noted in 1815 that ether had a similar effect. It was first used as an aid to surgery by Crawford Long (1815–78) in the USA. A dentist, William Thomas Morton (1819–68) demonstrated ether anaesthesia at Massachusetts General Hospital in 1846. In Britain, the first operation under ether anaesthesia was performed at University College Hospital, London, late in 1846 by Robert Liston (1794–1847). He was a surgeon noted for his speed and dexterity, necessary attributes in pre-anaesthetic days. His comment was 'this Yankee dodge beats mesmerism hollow'.[14]

Joseph Lister, later Lord Lister (1827–1912), was present as a student at the operation. When he became Professor of Clinical Surgery at Glasgow in 1860, he engaged in research into suppuration in wounds and concluded that the cause was not the noxious air in hospitals but something carried in the air. When his attention was directed to the work of Louis Pasteur (1822–95) on microbial fermentation causing the souring of wine and milk, he realised that this was the key to the problem. From it came his paper 'On the Antiseptic System of Treatment in Surgery' in the *British Medical Journal* (1868) and a new era of safety in surgery had begun.

The West Riding Asylum at Wakefield was directed from 1866 to 1875 by Dr (later Sir) James Crichton-Browne (1840–1938) who instituted a series of research reports, to which such subsequently famous doctors as John Hughlings Jackson, (Sir) Clifford Allbutt and (Sir) Thomas Lauder Brunton contributed. Dr (later Sir) David Ferrier (1843–1928) had been a fellow-student of Crichton-Browne at Edinburgh and visited him in 1873. Following that visit, he began research on faradic stimulation of the brain, working on vertebrates up to the monkey. From this research he was able to show the localisation of function in the brain. Lord Lister was his colleague at King's College, London, and Ferrier followed Listerian precautions against sepsis. This convinced him that brain surgery was feasible and he declared this in his Marshall Hall Oration at the Royal College of Physicians of London in 1883, and in 1884 (Sir) Rickman Godlee (1848–1925), nephew and biographer of Lister, removed a cerebral tumour which had been correctly localised by application of Ferrier's teaching. Ferrier and Hughlings Jackson were present at the operation.

Before that, after the publication of Ferrier's treatise *The Functions of the Brain* in 1876, (Sir) William McEwen (1848–1924), who had been house surgeon to Lister's pupil and successor in Glasgow, had removed a brain tumour in 1878 and had operated for the relief of subdural haemorrhage in 1879.

When Burckhardt published his work in 1890, there was such an outcry because a psychiatrist was performing surgical operations that he was discouraged and went no further. Apart from a report on mental patients in Finland by Puusepp, protégé of the Russian physiologist von Bechterev, in 1912, nothing more happened in the surgical treatment of mental illness until the 1930s.

At the international Congress of Neurology in London in 1935, Fulton and Jacobsen reported on the results of operating on the brains of chimpanzees which were experimentally made subject to attacks of sham rage. They found, as Burckhardt had, that interruption of the connections of the frontal lobes produced docility. Professor Egas Moniz, a neuropsychiatrist of Lisbon, was impressed by this fact and broached to Fulton the possibility of operating on human patients, but received no encouragement. Nevertheless, when he returned to Lisbon he persuaded his neurosurgical colleague Almeida Lima, who had been trained by Sir Hugh Cairns at Oxford, to operate on the connections between the frontal lobes and the thalamus, which is a large subcortical collection of gray matter (cells) mediating feeling. Alcohol injections proved useless but interruption of the nerve fibres (white matter) by blind cutting produced amelioration of the aggressive behaviour of chronic schizophrenics. The operation therefore became known as leucotomy, from the Greek words for white and cutting. In the USA, where it was taken up by W. Freeman, Professor of Neurology at George Washington University, and his neurosurgical colleague J.W. Watts, it acquired the name lobotomy.[15,16]

Because of spectacular results in some very disturbed patients, especially those who had not responded to convulsive therapy or insulin coma therapy, the operation gained widespread acceptance in the USA and in Europe. It was, however, not without its opponents, who included not only experienced psychiatrists but such disparate authorities as the Catholic Church and the Communist Party of the Soviet Union. In the early stages after operation, patients tended to show the symptoms of frontal lobe damage — restlessness, uninhibited social behaviour, lack of foresight, silliness, tactlessness. In most cases the grosser features cleared up as post-operative swelling in the operation area subsided. In other cases apathy and emotional blunting set in because the operation incision, which was made at a site not too exactly measured, was misplaced. When it was established that the lesion was best placed in the lower inner (inferomedial) quadrant of the frontal lobe, new approaches and modified operations were devised.

In 1954, for instance, Freeman approached the undersurface of the frontal lobe by pushing an ice-pick through the frontal sinus at the root of the nose while the patient was rendered unconscious by ECT. This violation of surgical principles ended his partnership with Watts. Grantham made his approach from the upper surface of the skull with needle electrodes, visualised by x-ray, and produced the required lesion by electrocoagulation. Knight in 1965 reported the results of implants of the isotope yttrium-90 which produced temporary low-grade radiation.

In 1961, Tooth and Newton reported to the Ministry of Health on operations on 10,365 patients which had been carried out between 1942 and 1954. They concluded that 41% of patients could be classified as recovered, 13% had made a social recovery and 25% were unchanged. Thirty per cent of the schizophrenic patients were able to leave hospital.[17]

The best results were obtained in patients of previously good personality who suffered from intractable depression, chronic anxiety or persistent obsessive-compulsive symptoms. The best authorities held that the illness must have been severe and crippling for at least two years and must have resisted non-invasive treatment methods such as ECT, medication and psychotherapy before leucotomy should be considered. Patients of poor personality structure exhibiting such features as apathy or shallow shifting moods and immature behaviour were among those who did badly. Results in schizophrenia were variable and those patients with long histories of apathy and deteriorated performance did not do so well. Patients with positive symptoms of aggression and mood change did better. Neglect of standard techniques of psychiatric rehabilitation after operation contributed to poor results. The advent of the neuroleptic and antidepressant drugs reduced the numbers of treatment-resistant patients and the need for leucotomy.

In 1949, Spiegel and Wycis of Temple University, Philadelphia, described a stereotactic instrument which, working in three dimensions with the head in a fixed plane, enabled the surgeon to locate the operation area in the brain precisely. Brain scanners, electrical recordings and x-rays increase the accuracy. Thus, nowadays psychosurgery is carried out only in a few centres where there are experienced teams of psychiatrists, psychologists and neurosurgeons. It has recently been remarked that such is their expertise in the assessment and alternative treatment of the patients

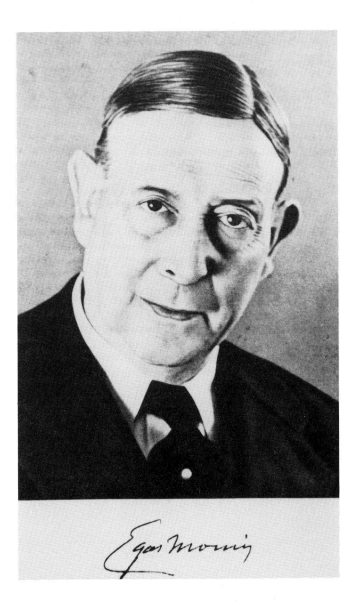

*Professor Egas Moniz*

referred that only a small percentage now actually proceed to operation.

Another application of surgery in the treatment of mental disease was in the eradication of possible sources of toxaemia. Acute toxic-confusional psychoses and infective-exhaustive states resulting from severe bacterial infection were well recognised, but hidden foci of infection as a cause for chronic mental illness were also postulated. Sir William Arbuthnot Lane (1856–1943) the eminent surgeon and Ilya Metchnikoff (1845–1916) the Russian biologist and Nobel prize-winner had both, in the first two decades of the 20th century, taught that toxins absorbed as a result of intestinal stasis were the cause of many of the ills of man. In 1932 the *Journal of Mental Science* published a special number on 'Sinusitis in Mental Disorder' in which Dr T. C. Graves of Birmingham with his collaborators Drs Watson-Williams and Pickworth described their findings of 818 cases of nasopharyngeal sepsis in 1000 psychiatric patients examined over a period of five years. 880 of them had had a puncture and wash-out of the nasal sinuses. In the same issue other psychiatrists expressed difficulty in accepting their theories in full and an editorial in the *British Medical Journal* of 31st December suggested that reciprocal enthusiasm in a team 'may reinforce each other's credence in an hypothesis beyond the customary standard of proof'.

## References

1. Annotation (1940). *Lancet*; **ii**:754.
2. *Board of Control Reports* (1934). Mapperley Hospital.
3. Critchley M. (1979). *The Divine Banquet of the Brain*. New York: Raven Press.
4. L'Etang H. (1980). *Fit to Lead*. London: Heinemann.
5. Martin J.P. (1972). Conquest of general paralysis. *British Medical Journal*; **3**:159.
6. Rinkel M., Himwich H.E., eds. (1959). *Insulin Treatment in Psychiatry*. New York: Philosophical Library.
7. Wilson I.G.H. (1937). *A Study of Hypoglycaemic Shock Treatment in Schizophrenia* (Board of Control Report). London: HMSO.
8. Bourne H. (1953). The insulin myth *Lancet*; **ii**:964.
9. Ackner B., Harris A., Oldham A.J. (1957). Insulin treatment of schizophrenia: a controlled study. *Lancet;* **i**:607.
10. Sim M. (1974). *Guide to Psychiatry*. Edinburgh and London: Churchill Livingstone.
11. Kalinowsky L.B., Hoch P. (1961). *Somatic Treatment in Psychiatry*. Philadelphia: Grune & Stratton.

12. Sargant W. (1967). *The Unquiet Mind*. London: Heinemann.
13. Impastato D.J. (1960). The story of the first electroshock treatment. *American Journal of Psychiatry*; **116**:1113.
14. Guthrie D. (1945). A History of Medicine, p.302 London: Nelson.
15. Fulton J.F. (1952). *Frontal Lobotomy and Affective Behaviour; The Sherrington Lectures*. University Press of Liverpool.
16. Freeman W., Watts J.W. (1942 and 1950). *Psychosurgery*. Springfield, Ill: Charles C. Thomas.
17. Tooth G.C., Newton M.P. (1961). Leucotomy in England and Wales 1942–1954:Reports on Public Health and Medical Subjects No.104. London: HMSO.

# CHAPTER 5

# *Medicinal Treatment*

The use of medicines, simple or compound, organic or inorganic, started in prehistoric days. The earliest would be plant extracts and mineral waters. From Greek mythology comes the story of Melampus. The twin, some say triplet, daughters of Proetus, King of Argos, were visited by madness because they rejected the worship of

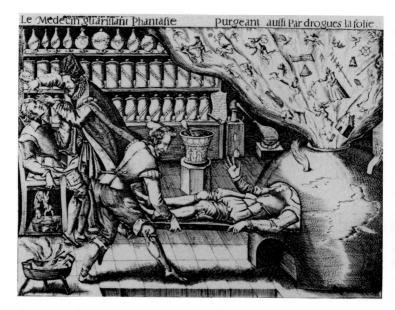

*A seventeenth century print showing the physician curing fantasy and purging madness with drugs*

Dionysius and insulted the goddess Hera. Melampus, who was reputed to have treated Hercules, undertook to cure them in exchange for one-third of the kingdom for himself, and another third for his brothers. Having noted that goats which ate hellebore were violently purged, he gave the plant extract to the girls in milk and then made them run until they were exhausted. After undergoing purifiying rites at the temple of Artemis in Arcadia, they recovered. Thus purgation as a treatment of mental illness was established. The rationale could be either the evacuation of the poisons, bad humours or evil spirits which were causing the illness, or the production of physical prostration to be followed by revival to a new healthy life. The hellebore which Melampus used was the black variety, *Helleborus niger*, the Christmas rose (or, 'specific of Anticyra', where it grew). It was in use until the eighteenth century. Thomas Willis prescribed it for melancholy. *Veratrum album*, the false or white hellebore, is also a violent purgative and was advocated for mania and epilepsy. No doubt the overactivity of the manic patient was reduced by exhaustion.

Another early specific was nepenthes. Homer referred to it in the Odyssey as a drug of Egyptian origin, capable of banishing grief or trouble. Gerard thought it could be borage.

## The herbals and the herbalists

A knowledge of plants and their medicinal actions was necessary, not only for physicians who were comparatively few, but also for those priests, monks, wise men and wise women who also undertook the care of the sick. This knowledge was gathered together and published by interested parties. In about 300 BC, Theophrastus, pupil and successor of Aristotle as President of the Lyceum, wrote a *History of Plants* in which he described 500 plants with curative properties. Pliny the Elder (AD 23–79) in his encyclopaedic *Historia Naturalis* mentions 1000. His contemporary Dioscorides (AD 40–90), a native of Cicilia and probably an army doctor, wrote *De Materia Medica*. His influence can be seen in the Anglo-Saxon *Leech Book of Bald* and he was still quoted by William Turner (1508–68) in his *New Herball* of 1551.

The most famous English herbalist is John Gerard (1545–1612). He published his *Herball* in 1597 and in it he drew on his experience as a barber-surgeon and as a gardener.

Nicholas Culpeper (1616–54) wrote *The English Physician Enlarged* in 1651 and described 300 native medicinal plants. He was very attracted by the Doctrine of Signatures which held that a specific mark or appearance of a plant indicated its therapeutic use. For example, the yellow celandine was good for jaundice and the walnut for head injuries: the shell for wounds of the skull and the kernel for the brain. Gerard also followed this train of thought when he recommended a purgation of black hellebore 'for all those that are troubled with black choler and molested by melancholy'.

In addition to hellebore and borage, the following were prescribed for melancholy or depression: bugloss steeped in wine 'comfermeth and conserveth the mind'; chrysanthemum 'also it is good for such as be melancholick, sad, pensive and without speech' — Gerard); lemon balm; the saffron crocus (*C. sativus*) used by Mongols, Greeks, Romans and Arabs to provoke merriment; the day lily (*'Hemerocallis fulva'*); eglantine or sweetbriar; and the scent of dry roses or rosewater (Robert Burton: *The Anatomy of Melancholy*, 1621).

For epilepsy or the falling sickness there were marsh marigold, carnation or gillyflower, the male paeony *(Leech Book of Bald)*, and heartsease (*Viola tricolor*).

Sundry psychotropic herbs included acanthus, a mollifying herb; alyssum or madwort for abating rage; marigold 'draweth out of ye heed wikkid hirores' (humours); honesty or moonwort, Chaucer's lunarie tansy, for 'warming and drying the brain and opening the stoppings of the same' (Gerard); and scull cap against hydrophobia.

Bad humours could be driven out or warded off with periwinkle and rosemary. White and yellow fumiterre (*Corydalis bulbosa*) were grown by Gerard in his own garden. The smoke drove off evil spirits. Lobelia, still used in a tincture in the twentieth century, relieved spasms. The leaves of yarrow in the nose relieved the pain of megrim or migraine (Gerard). Another herb which survived in tincture form and in a mixture with potassium bromide well into this century was valerian. It was prescribed for the very common anxiety and mild depressive neurosis. Its early use for hysteria was explained on the grounds that the wandering uterus which was causing the symptoms did not like the smell of this herb and would return to its proper location. From the herbals, we can discern the medicines favoured for neurotic symptoms: meadowsweet, water-mint and vervian; catmint tea, lime flowers, lavender, rue for nervous headaches; camomile tea as a sedative, 'to comfort the braine smel to

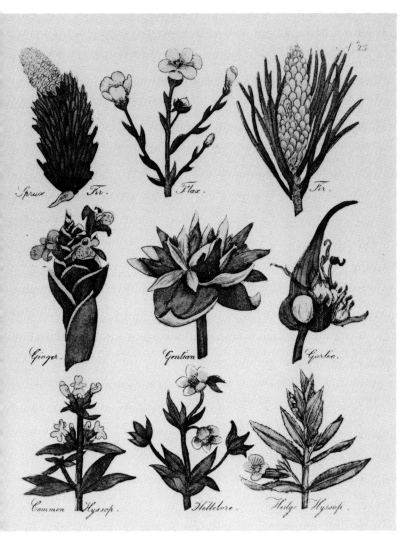

*A plate from Culpeper's* Complete Herbal *showing hellebore*

camomil'; gentian and motherwort as tonics; thyme for the vapours
and white bryony for hysteria; sweet marjoram for a sexual nerve
sedative; powdered betony with wine to be taken 'at the tyme the
fere cometh' (Peter Treveris: *Grete Herball*, 1526). [1,2,3,4,5]

William Withering (1741–99), a Midland physician, applied the herb lore of an old Staffordshire woman by treating congestive heart failure with a preparation of foxglove (*Digitalis purpurea*). In his account of the foxglove and some of its medical uses, he described two cases of delirium in which heart failure was producing defective circulation in the brain and which were relieved by his treatment.[6] Others did not differentiate this organic confusional state from mental illness and used digitalis for all cases. As large doses produced nausea, vomiting and diarrhoea, it was in line with the debilitating treatments then in vogue. The other effects of slowing the pulse of the excited patient and producing an increased output of urine, thereby being credited with reducing excess water in the brain, were also welcomed.

## The narcotics

These comprise henbane (*Hyoscyamus niger*), mandrake or mandragora, belladonna (*Atropa belladonna*), Indian hemp (*Cannabis indica*) and poppy (*Papaver somniferum*). Their properties are to have an effect on alertness or arousal, on mood and on the perception of pain. Thus in small doses they can have a euphoriant action and in slightly higher dosage an analgesic effect. Sleep can be induced, or stupor, which is a state in which consciousness is dulled and stimuli are not attended to. When Iago is planning to inflict severe mental pain on Othello, Shakespeare has him say:

'Not poppy nor mandragora
Nor all the drowsy syrups of the world,
Shall ever medicine thee to that sweet sleep
Which thou Ow'dst yesterday.'

Their usefulness in relieving pain, insomnia and distress is counterbalanced by the drawback that with continued use they can produce dependence, tolerance and addiction: increasing amounts are needed for relief and withholding them results in indescribable suffering.

Henbane was recommended by Aretaeus in the second century. Andrew Boorde (1490–1549), in his *Breviary of Healthe*, said that it caused 'frantickness' or toxic delirium in modern terms. The active principle in henbane is hyoscine or scopolamine. With morphine it has been used in 'twilight sleep' in obstetrics and as an emergency tranquilliser in states of excitement.

Mandrake is a root. Because of its occasional resemblance to a human body, the fanciful believed that it had a life of its own and when dug up it would shriek with pain. Furthermore, those who heard the shriek (or squeak) would be sorely affected. Therefore, the root gatherers, after prayers to Apollo and Aesculapius, would tie the root to the collar of a dog and let the animal pull it out while they retired to a safe distance. Pliny wrote that patients would chew mandrake and belladonna as an anaesthetic before surgery.

Cannabis (hashish) was introduced into medicine by Arab physicians and was known to Avicenna in the tenth century. Its production of a mood of detachment and unnatural perception in its users commended it for the treatment of depression and emotional disorder, although the results were poor. Nevertheless, cannabis retained a place in the pharmacopoeia until late in the nineteenth century, according to Daniel Hack Tuke in his *Chapters in the History of the Insane in the British Isles* (1882).

'Of all the remedies which it has pleased Almighty God to give to man to relieve his suffering, none is so universal and so efficacious as opium.' (Thomas Sydenham, 1624–89). Opium was made from the juice of the poppy and seems to have come from the Levant. The name Tinctura Thebaica (of Thebes) would indicate an origin in Egypt and from what we know of its properties it is more likely that it, rather than Gerard's borage, can be identified as Homer's nepenthes. References to its narcotic effects abound in texts ancient, medieval and recent. Celsus (23 BC–AD 50) recommended a decoction of poppies for insomnia. Bartholomaeus Anglicus in the thirteenth century directed that the patient's temples and forehead should be anointed with the juice of the poppy for 'the frenesie'. Five centuries later, the great Italian reformer Vincenzo Chiarugi (1759–1820) treated patients who resisted oral medication by inunction with powdered opium in a simple ointment. John Brown (1735–88) advocated supportive and stimulating treatment rather than bleeding and purging and used opium and alcohol freely. The rise of moral treatment caused a lessening of interest in medication, but in the last three decades of the nineteenth centruy, opium and its alkaloids — morphine, codeine, thebaine — were again being advocated for the treatment of mania by Sir Thomas Clouston, father of the author of *A Lunatic at Large*, and in a letter to the *British Medical Journal* in 1881 Dr William Murrell quoted various authorities, including De Quincey, saying that a moderate intake of opium was not harmful and calling for further information on the possibility of its use.

Before the 1940s Nepenthe, a commercial aqueous extract of the alkaloids of opium, was in use as a sedative and hypnotic, and Tincture of Opium, the original alcoholic extract known as laudanum, was still put up with potassium bromide and chloral hydrate in the mixture known as Three Fifteens: fifteen minims of the tincture with fifteen grains of each of the others per dose. Paracelsus (1493–1541) claimed that his laudanum was made from gold leaf and dissolved pearls, but its resemblance to the opiate was too strong for his deception to endure. The combination of opium and alcohol, originally devised by the Arabs, enhanced its appeal and its tendency to produce addiction.

*Rauwolfia serpentina* — the name was bestowed on it in 1703 to honour Leonard Rauwolf of Augsburg who described it in 1582 — is a herb used as a sedative for thousands of years in India. It is said to have also been known to Avicenna and to the Chinese. A Portuguese book published in Goa in 1563 called it 'Primum et Laudatissimum remedium' but it was not introduced into Western medicine until the 1940s.

## Chemistry and the development of psychopharmacology

The earliest chemists were the Arabs, and from North Africa and Moorish Spain their knowledge diffused into Europe. Gabir Ibn Hayan (AD 702–765) devised the processes of distillation, filtration and sublimation and made aqua regia or nitric acid. Alcohol, alkali, aldehyde, alembic, alchemy, camphor, senna, are all words from the Arabic. In the sixteenth century, interest started to deviate from alchemy, with its search for the philosopher's stone for the transmutation of base metals into gold, to chemistry which investigated the properties of elements and their compounds. Although Paracelsus was very interested in alchemy and mysticism and expressed himself obscurely and combatively, he did propose some insights and improvements in chemistry and pharmacy.

Andreas Libavius (1540–1616) wrote a lucid account of medical chemistry, *Alchymia recognita*, in 1597 but it was in the nineteenth century that the first discoveries forming the foundation of modern psychopharmacological treatments were made.

Morphine was isolated in 1803 by Wilhelm Friedrich Adam

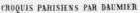

CROQUIS PARISIENS PAR DAUMIER

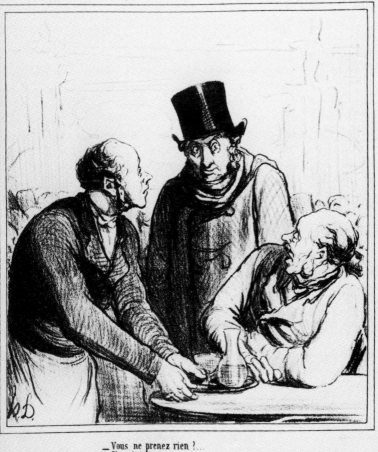

_ Vous ne prenez rien ?...
_ Non, j'ai peur....
_ Allons, un grog au laudanum !...

*Nineteenth century treatment of anxiety neurosis*

Setürner (1783–1841), a pharmacist's assistant from Paderborn, and hyoscine was synthesised by Schmidt in 1888. Lithium was discovered in petalite by Arfvedson in 1818. The synthesis of urea by Wohler in 1828 destroyed the theory that the formation of biological substances required a vital force. Justus von Liebig (1803–73) synthesised chloroform in 1831 and chloral hydrate in 1832. The latter was used by Liebreich in 1869 as a sedative and hypnotic, because he thought, mistakenly, that it released chloroform in the body. It was administered intravenously by Ore of Lyons in 1872. Chloral is still favoured today as a hynotic in elixir form or in more elegant solid preparations.

Potassium bromide, known since the 1830s, was widely used as a sedative, a hypnotic and an anticonvulsant. Accumulation of the drug in the body could give rise to bromism, a state of toxic confusion which could be mistaken for a worsening of the illness and would cause the patient to require admission to hospital for what started as a mild condition. Evelyn Waugh's *The Ordeal of Gilbert Pinfold* is the description of bromide intoxication.

Barbituric acid was prepared by von Baeyer in 1862. The connection with St Barbara is a matter for speculation. The first barbiturate hypnotic, Veronal, was produced by Fischer and von Mering in 1903. The name commemorates a visit to Italy. Phenobarbitone, an indifferent sedative but still a useful anticonvulsant in epilepsy, followed in 1912. A soluble and injectable barbiturate, somnifaine, was the basis of Kläsi's continuous narcosis in 1920. Amylobarbitone in 1923 and quinalbarbitone and pentobarbitone in 1930 became popular for the relief of anxiety and insomnia because they were of quick action and short duration. In chronic neurotic states they could become drugs of habituation and in some cases of addiction, and overdoses could be fatal. With the introduction of the benzodiazepines, they are much less used. The campaign against the prescribing of barbiturates is motivated not only because safe and effective alternatives now exist, but also in order to reduce their availability to drug abusers who resort to criminal activity to obtain them.

Iminodibenzyl, the basis of the first of the thymoleptics (mood modifiers), was synthesised by Thiele and Holzinger in 1898, and phenothiazine, the forerunner of the neuroleptics or major tranquillisers, by Bernsthen in 1883.

Paraldehyde is a bitter-tasting liquid of characteristic and penetrating odour. It is very efficient in calming states of excitement and over-activity, in promoting sleep and, by injection, in terminating the repeated convulsions of status epilepticus. Its free use in mental hospitals advertised itself by the smell which met one at the ward door if not at the front door. It was first used by Covello in 1882, although Wiedenbusch had made it in 1829. In his Presidential

Address to the Royal Medico-Psychological Association in 1958, Dr L.C. Cook was describing the changes wrought in Bexley Mental Hospital by the physical treatments and mentioned that during 1938 the hospital used 1430 lb of paraldehyde and 273 lb of chloral hydrate, and how much those figures had been reduced. Sulphonal was another powerful tranquilliser prepared from acetone in 1886 and in use until the middle of this century. Like paraldehyde it has been superseded by the newer products of the pharmaceutical industry.[7,8]

## The neuroleptic drugs

The term neuroleptic (having an effect on the neurones) was proposed by Delay and Deniker in 1955 to describe those tranquillising drugs which differed from previously known tranquillisers and sedatives in two ways. They had a direct effect on the symptoms — delusions, hallucinations, disorders of mood and behaviour — of the psychoses and they had a tendency to produce neurological symptoms which were reversible when the drug was reduced in dose or withdrawn. The desirable antipsychotic qualities had not been exhibited by any of the drugs previously available. The undesirable neurological symptoms — spasmodic and continuous disorders of muscle tone (dystonia), abnormal movements (dyskinesia) and uncontrolled restlessness (akathesia) and the tremors, rigidity and the salivation of Parkinson's disease — were those which had been seen in the 1920s in the patients whose brains had been damaged in the epidemic of encephalitis lethargica.

Chlorpromazine, the first of the phenothiazine derivatives, was synthesised in 1950 by Charpentier in the Rhône-Poulenc laboratories. At the time there was interest in artificial hibernation, a method of lowering the body's metabolism to reduce shock during surgical operations. Laborit devised a 'lytic cocktail' of pethidine, which resembles morphine, and promethazine, which is an antihistamine and a precursor of chlorpromazine, the third ingredient. The last-named produced in warm-blooded animals the conditions which occurred in the hibernation of cold-blooded animals. Laborit predicted that if it produced a state of ataraxia — freedom of the mind from pain or passion as desired by the Stoics — it would be useful in psychiatry. The cocktail was tried on manic patients at the Val de Grâce Military Hospital in Paris and the results were interesting but not spectacular.

Delay and Deniker then tried chlorpromazine alone and in higher doses. Manic excitement, agitation, aggression and delusional thinking in schizophrenics were relieved and therapeutic contact was more readily achieved. About this, Deniker says 'It was supported by the sudden great interest of the nursing personnel, who had always been reserved about innovations'. Delay and Deniker reported their first results in 1952.[9] Research into phenothiazine compounds was stimulated and there followed such drugs as promazine and thioridazine with weaker tranquillising effects, and others such as perphenazine with stronger antipsychotic properties, and trifluoperazine with an activating effect on withdrawn patients.

*Rauwolfia serpentina* returned to western medicine from India, when papers by Gupta in 1943 and Hakim in 1953 were noted. Of several alkaloids isolated from it in the CIBA laboratories, reserpine was found to be the most active. It had a calming effect on states of agitation and excitement, relieved psychotic symptoms in schizophrenia and lowered blood pressure. The main drawback was its tendency to produce severe depression and, because of this and the proliferation of other neuroleptics, its use declined.[10]

The success of these compounds stimulated pharmaceutical research and the objective was to produce tailor-made drugs with predictable biological properties. In the late 1950s and early 1960s Janssen Laboratories in Belgium produced a series known as the butyrophenones, of which haloperidol (1959) is the most widely used. Benperidol (1965) has been used specifically for patients with disorders of sexual impulse control and droperidol (1963) gives rapid temporary control of extreme agitation and is also a most useful auxiliary in anaesthesia, producing calmness and reducing post-operative shock.[9]

The Danish firm of Lundbeck explored the possibilities of a new chemical group, the thioxanthenes. Clopenthixol (introduced in 1959) and flupenthixol (1963) have also proved to be valuable neuroleptics. The latter drug is interesting because in doses too small to relieve psychosis it is effective in some cases of mild depression.[9]

There have always been acute recoverable cases of schizophrenia. Other patients have made a partial or social recovery enabling them to live without institutional care, although exhibiting some disability. The chronic schizophrenics requiring continued care and shelter have constituted the bulk of mental hospital populations and remained a challenge to medical and nursing ingenuity. The recent physical and drug treatments made it possible to discharge from hospital patients who would otherwise require in-patient care. They could be maintained in the community provided that drug treatment was continued on an out-patient or day-patient basis. That proviso unfortunately could not be guaranteed. Many patients — and the many includes non-psychiatric patients — cannot be relied on to take their drugs regularly. Failure to continue treatment would lead to a relapse, necessitating re-admission to hospital or resulting in a drifting away from regular supervision. A great improvement in the defaulting was brought about when it became possible to administer neuroleptics in a long-acting form by intramuscular injection. A depot is formed in the tissues from which the drug is slowly absorbed. Thus, with one dose given at intervals of one to four weeks, a continuous drug intake can be achieved. The control of symptoms and the regular contact with medical and nursing staff which this regime necessitates have therapeutic benefits, which, to judge from patient compliance, far outweigh any dislike of repeated injections. Fluphenazine enanthate (1963) was followed by fluphenazine decanoate in 1965. Other drugs for depot injection are fluspiriline (1968) and flupenthixol (1967).

## The antidepressant drugs

These have been called thymoleptic (having an effect on mood). The word 'depression' is used in psychiatry in two ways. It is the name of a state of feeling of misery, sadness, lack of pleasure, which is a symptom in mental illness. It is also the name of a group of illnesses in which, in addition to the depressive symptom, there can be anxiety or morbid fear, tension, irritability, loss of interest and drive, impaired concentration, retardation of thought and action, feelings of guilt, delusions of guilt or disease or disaster, loss of appetite, loss of sleep, contemplation of or an attempt at suicide.

In 1927, Gordon Alles (1901–1963) synthesised amphetamine as a substitute for ephedrine in the treatment of asthma. One form of amphetamine, the dextro-isomer, was found to be a powerful stimulant of brain activity. It prolonged wakefulness, increased alertness and relieved fatigue. It was used in the German Army and in the Royal Air Force in the Second World War. The Japanese used the methyl derivative. As dexamphetamine also produced euphoria, it was tried in depressive illnesses. The stimulant effect was too dis-

turbing for many patients. Therefore, a sedative, sodium amylobarbitone, was added. The combination, because of the colour and
shape of the tablet, was dubbed 'purple heart'. Some patients with
mild depression and tension were helped but it did not relieve the
severe retarded depressions, the classic melancholia. Its euphoriant
action led to addiction in some patients and to great popularity with
the drug-abusing section of the population.

Antihistamine drugs were the starting point in the development of
one class of antidepressants as well as the neuroleptics. In 1950, the
Swiss firm of Geigy asked Dr Roland Kuhn of Münsterlingen to try
one of their antihistamines, with the code number G22150, as a
hypnotic. It was not satisfactory but there were indications of mild
antipsychotic activity which the makers did not follow up. When the
action of chlorpromazine became known, the drug was tried again
with no better results. Another of the series with a side-chain similar
to that of chlorpromazine was coded G22355. Kuhn tried it on about
300 patients with varying diagnosis. Early in 1956 it was tried on
three patients with endogenous (retarded) depression and its antidepressant action was obvious. The results in 40 cases were reported
to a small audience at the Second International Congress of
Psychiatry at Zurich in 1957.[11] G22355 was imipramine, the first of
the tricyclic compounds, so called because of their chemical config-
uration. From it were derived desipramine, trimipramine and
chlormipramine, in attempts to improve on its efficacy and its speed
of action. Chlormipramine was advocated not only for the treatment
of depression but also for obsessive-compulsive neurosis. Amitrip-
tyline was introduced in 1959, protriptyline, nortriptyline and but-
riptyline being later developments. Several others have come along
in the following 20 years. They include tetracyclic compounds and
others which are claimed to have fewer side-effects and swifter
action. These drugs have revolutionised the treatment of the depressive illnesses, relieving much suffering and shifting the locus of
treatment from the ward to the consulting room. They are not
effective in some of the severely depressed patients and therefore,
while reducing the need for ECT, have not rendered it wholly
unnecessary.

The forerunner of a different group of antidepressant drugs was,
like imipramine, tried as a neuroleptic and, also like imipramine
escaped being discarded as useless. Iproniazid was a drug developed
by Hoffman-La Roche for the treatment of tuberculosis. It would

have been discontinued because of its side-effects had not one group of clinicians insisted on its superiority in the treatment of bone tuberculosis. One of the side-effects noted in tuberculosis patients was euphoria and elation, but nobody thought of it as an antidepressant. Trials suggested by the success of chlorpromazine in 1953 showed it was disappointing as a tranquilliser. Experiments in 1956 showed that animals treated with reserpine and iproniazid became hyperalert and hyperactive. It was only in 1957, when Dr Nathan Kline of New York and his colleagues began treating depressed patients in private practice with iproniazid alone, that its value was recognised. The eagerness with which it was taken up following the publication of their results showed how great was the need for an effective drug treatment of depressive illness.[9] Enthusiasm for the newcomer became dampened when cases of jaundice appeared in some of the patients treated. The same thing had been observed in some receiving chorpromazine. Of course, the drugs were blamed. Little notice was taken of the fact that it was a time when virus hepatitis, of which jaundice is a symptom, was also present in the population.

The biochemical action of iproniazid was found to be that it prevented the action of any enzyme, an oxidase which breaks down amine compounds in the body. These compounds are depleted in depression. Their concentration is built up again when their normal breakdown is reduced. So runs a simplified account of the process. Thus iproniazid was described as a monoamine oxidase inhibitor, MAOI for short. Several other MAOI were developed, of which isocarboxazid, phenelzine and tranylcypromine are the present-day survivors. Dr William Sargant and his colleagues at St Thomas' Hospital, London, showed that the MAOI are less effective in the retarded or melancholic type of depression but produce improvement in neurotic and atypical depressions, that is, in those conditions in which tension, irritability and anxiety are more prominent and bouts of depression are irregular in incidence and duration.

All effective drugs have side-effects. The neuroleptics have the neurological side-effects previously mentioned. The tricyclic antidepressant drugs produce a dry mouth and constipation and, in some sensitive patients, a drop in blood pressure or difficulty in passing water are limiting side-effects. In 1961 and 1962, there came scattered reports that some patients on MAOI had attacks in which the blood pressure rose acutely producing a severe and painful headache and collapse. When these reports were collated in a letter to *The Lancet* by Dr (later Professor) Barry Blackwell, they evoked a communication from a hospital pharmacist (G.E.F. Rowe) in Nottingham detailing the two attacks which his wife had had after eating cheese. Detective work by Dr Blackwell confirmed the link with cheese and he followed it up with research to elucidate the nature of the disturbing ingredient. This was found to be tyramine which, in susceptible individuals, was concentrated in the absence of the oxidase to a level which produced the acute rise in blood pressure. Other articles of diet containing an unacceptable level of tyramine were found to be yeast extract (Bovril, Oxo, Marmite), red wine, especially Chianti, and strong beers including lager. The pods of broad beans contain an amine related to tyramine, as also do some varieties of pickled herring. In addition, the narcotics morphine and pethidine, amphetamines, ephedrine and similar pressor drugs could produce the hypertensive reaction. Such limitations would have rendered the drugs unacceptable had not their advantages outweighed the disadvantages. The MAOI have produced relief of neurotic depressions which no other drug combination has done.

## The anxiolytic drugs

Fear, with its feeling of sickening apprehension and its bodily accompaniments of dry mouth, cold sweat, palpitations, stomach churning, tremors etc., is the biological reaction to a life-threatening situation. In psychiatric parlance, anxiety is the fear reaction displaced into situations which are not life-threatening, but which evoke it by actual or symbolic resemblance to the original stress or stresses. Therefore, medicinal substances which dissolve or wash away the symptoms of anxiety and render the afflicted person more comfortable have always been sought. Reference has already been made to the use of opium, bromides and the barbiturates. They were not ideal and not wholly successful. Mild states of anxiety were relieved by dulling the senses and tension was relieved by removing the inhibitions and self-awareness imposed by the higher levels of mind through the higher nervous centres. The same effects are produced by alcohol and, as with alcohol, the bigger doses called for by more severe anxiety states resulted in impairment of consciousness and motor skills, and toxic effects in organs other than the nervous system. Prolonged use led to abuse, addiction and personality deterioration. This undesirable reputation is one reason why relatives, friends and nonpsychiatric doctors will nag patients to stop taking their psychotropic medication long before they have recovered, making them feel guilty and increasing their distress. They do not appreciate that the newer drugs are the products of rational research, experiments and observation, that they are more effective in non-toxic doses and that they are non-addictive. They are more effective because they act on the biochemical systems which service the neuronal circuits mediating the symptoms of anxiety, tension and depression. Concentration and alertness are improved when the patient's attention is on the task in hand and is not distracted by inappropriate signals. Continued dependency is not the effect of the drug. It is due to the prolonged natural history of psychiatric disorders and the delayed response to or failure of adjuvant treatment.

The success of the sulphonamides and of penicillin as antibacterial agents led to a search for compounds which could kill organisms not affected by penicillin. One compound, synthesised by Berger and Bradley in 1946, was found to produce a reversible paralysis of muscles and a quietening effect in experimental animals. They called the effect tranquillisation and the compound mephenesin. Clinically it proved useful in producing muscular relaxation in light anaesthesia and shortly after that it was shown to allay anxiety without clouding consciousness and it induced a feeling of relaxation in tense and anxious patients. The disadvantages were its short duration of action and its lack of potency. Further development led to the discovery of meprobamate by Ludwig in 1950. Its sedative action lasted about eight times as long as mephenesin and it had a taming effect on vicious animals. When marketed under the name of Miltown, it became widely used in the USA, and to a lesser extent in Europe. Its value was in the treatment of anxiety states. The work of neurophysiologists showed that meprobamate acted on the thalamus and the limbic system of the brain. These are the structures lying below the cerebral cortex which were first proposed by Papez in 1937 as providing the neuronal circuits serving the mechanism of anxiety. This would explain the unsuitability of meprobamate in the treatment of the psychoses: it did not act on the brain area reached by the successful neuroleptics.

By the mid-1950s, psychopharmacological research was being vigorously pursued. In the New Jersey laboratories of Hoffman-La Roche, Dr Leo Sternbach resumed an interest in a group of compounds called heptoxdiazines. They were first known in 1891 and their structure was elucidated in 1924. Dr Sternbach was synthesising new members of the heptoxdiazines in the late 1930s when he was working at the University of Cracow. He chose them because there was available chemical information about them and further modifications could be made relatively easily. The results of screening for biological activity were disappointing. The last compound of the series, Ro 5-0690, was put aside in 1955, without being tested. When the laboratory was being tidied up in 1957, it was sent for pharmacological testing and was discovered to be more potent than meprobamate. Re-examination of its chemical structure identified it as a benzodiazepine. Hospital trials in 1958 showed it to have strong sedative properties and it produced ataxia and slurred speech in patients, which was a disappointment. Luckily, the Director of Biological Research decided to persist and offered the Ro 5-0690 to three clinicians for trials on out-patients, who are always more numerous than in-patients. Experience with meprobamate had shown that it was not always effective in severe anxiety states. The phenothiazines were apt to produce lassitude in these patients without stemming anxiety. The new drug, given in smaller doses than used in hospital, was found to be much more efficient than either and quite suitable for ambulant patients. Clinical trials were completed in 1959 and chlordiazepoxide, marketed as Librium, was released in 1960 and became one of the most widely used drugs in the world.[9]

The benzodiazepine formula could now be developed. Diazepam was synthesised by Dr Sternbach in 1959 and introduced into clinical practice in 1963 as Valium. For some patients it was a better tranquilliser than chlordiazepoxide. Pharmacological testing showed the benzodiazepines to have an anticonvulsant action but they are of no use in epilepsy, except that diazepam is the most efficient and safest drug for controlling the repeated fits in status epilepticus. Because of the wide margin between the therapeutic and toxic doses, they have also proved to be a safe treatment in delirium tremens. Other early benzodiazepines have been oxazepam, synthesised in Wyeth Laboratories in 1961, and nitrazepam, the hypnotic known as Mogadon. In the succeeding 20 years, other anxiolytics and hypnotics in the same series have been developed, although those mentioned have continued to hold their place in the psychiatric armamentarium.

## Lithium treatment

That painful scourge, gout, is marked by an excess of uric acid in the body. In 1859, A.B. Garrod used lithium salts in the treatment of gout because the urate was the most soluble of all urates. Although their toxic effects showed up from time to time, they were still in decreasing use in the fifth decade of this century when they were the subject of condemnatory reports. This was the unpropitious moment when Dr John Cade started the rehabilitation of lithium in therapeutics. In 1948 he was working in a small psychiatric hospital in Australia and was looking for evidence to test his hypothesis that the patient in mania was producing an internal intoxicating agent. Guinea-pigs injected with the urine of manic patients died from the toxic effect of urea. Uric acid enhanced the toxic effect. When Cade added lithium urate in order to get an idea of how much influence the uric acid had, he was surprised to find that the toxic effect was very much reduced. Suspecting the lithium component, he used lithium carbonate, with an even better result. Guinea-pigs which were usually timid, easily startled and overactive, became calm and placid. By an association of ideas, Cade connected the lithium effect with the manic patients who had provided the urine. As he knew that lithium had been used in medical treatment he was not worried, but he took several doses himself of lithium citrate and carbonate before giving them to patients. The first patient was a man aged 51 years who was in a deteriorated condition after exhibiting manic excitement continuously for five years. After five days there was an improvement, and after three weeks he moved to a convalescent ward. After 15 weeks he was discharged and returned to his old job. Six months later he was re-admitted having neglected to continue his medication. He improved in two weeks and was discharged in six weeks. A further nine manic patients in the same hospital showed the same favourable response. Lithium carbonate was found to be better tolerated than the citrate and established itself as the satisfactory treatment.[12]

Mania is one phase of the manic-depressive psychosis. Some patients have alternating phases of mania and depression, some have more attacks of mania than depression, some patients have depressions with only minimal signs of hypomania. A characteristic feature of the illness is the tendency to recur. Lithium treatment had become widely used in the 1950s. In Denmark, Baastrup and his co-workers in 1967[13] and again in 1970[14] published evidence that continued administration of lithium carbonate had a prophylactic effect and reduced or stopped the incidence of further attacks in manic-depressive patients. From this grew the practice of continued out-patient supervision with periodic measurement of the concentration of lithium in the blood. This indicated if the amount of lithium was reaching toxic levels or if it was too low to be of protective value. Thus, lithium carbonate is the first true psycho-prophylactic.

## Vitamin treatment

The deficiency diseases were known long before their prevention was understood and their rational treatment achieved. Daniel Whistler (1619–84), a friend of Samuel Pepys, and Francis Glisson (1597–1677) described rickets. Scurvy was described by Jacques de Vitry during the fifth crusade in the thirteenth century. The famous account, *A Treatise of the Scurvy*, was published in 1753 by James Lind (1716–94), a naval surgeon who cured and prevented the disease with lemon juice. Gaspar Casal (1679–1759) was a Spanish physician who described pellagra. Francesco Frapelli of Milan wrote on it in 1771, calling it Mal de la Rosa.[15] Sir Henry Holland (1788–1873), who was physician to Queen Caroline, William IV, Queen Victoria and Prince Albert, reported what he had seen of it in the peasants of Lombardy to the Medical and Chirurgical Society of London.[16] Jacobus Bontius (1592–1631) described beriberi, with which he became familiar in the Dutch East Indies. Nicholas Tulp (1593–1674), who never left Amsterdam and who is immortalised in Rembrandt's painting, described a case in a patient who returned from the East Indies.

Professor Szent-Gyorgyi (b. 1893), who synthesised ascorbic acid (vitamin C) in 1934 and was awarded a Nobel Prize in 1937, defined a vitamin as 'a substance which makes you ill if you don't eat it'! The existence of 'essential food factors' was suspected from the work of Lunin on diets in 1881, and Sir Frederick Gowland Hopkins (1861–1947) at Cambridge in 1906 showed that fat, carbohydrate and protein in pure form were not enough to maintain health. In Java, Christiaan Eijkman (1858–1930) was medical officer to a prison and became familiar with beriberi. When he fed chickens on the prisoners' diet, they too developed polyneuritis and dropsy, the symptoms of beriberi. This was in 1897. The substitution of unpolished rice for polished rice relieved it. The Japanese had abolished beriberi in their merchant ships in 1881 by doing this. If they had done it for their prisoners of war, there would have been less of the suffering described by de Wardener and Lennox (1947) who had to hide their clinical records in a cemetery until the end of the war.[17]

Eijkman was the first to produce a deficiency disease experimentally and he and Hopkins shared a Nobel Prize in 1929. Casimir Funk (b. 1884 in Warsaw) isolated the beriberi-preventing substance in 1912. It was he who called it a vitamine — shortened to vitamin by his assistant (Sir) Jack Drummond (1891–1952) — and it took its place as vitamin B. In 1926, Smith and Hendrick showed that there were two components, $B_1$ (thiamine) and $B_2$ which later research identified as a complex of which five components are of major importence — nicotinic acid, riboflavine, pyridoxine, folic acid and cyanocobalamin.

The B group comprises the vitamins which are of interest to the psychiatrist because they are necessary for the proper functioning of nerve cells. Their deficiency leads to organic disease of the brain with symptoms of mental illness.

Carl Wernicke (1848–1905) in 1881 described an illness in two chronic alcoholics and one patient with persistent vomiting with ocular palsies, ataxic gait and severe mental confusion. It was not until 1940 that similar lesions to theirs were demonstrated in the brains of thiamine-deficient pigeons. In the following year it was shown that thiamine relieved the palsies and improved the confusion in human subjects.

S.S. Korsakov (1854–1900) was Superintendent and Professor in the University of Moscow Psychiatric Clinic from 1892. In 1887 he had described a psychosis with polyneuritis, confusion and a profound disturbance of recent memory. A striking, but not essential, feature was a tendency to confabulation: the patient would fill the memory gaps with fabricated recollections which would be immediately forgotten and replaced with others if he were questioned again. It was observed in alcoholism chiefly but also in other conditions, such as cancer of the stomach, intractable vomiting and severe dietary deficiency. In the late 1930s, this led to a suspicion of thiamine deficiency and the administration of thiamine by injection was found to lessen the mental confusion, although the memory defects persisted. The work of de Wardener and Lennox in the prisoner of war camps of Singapore and Siam showed that Wernicke's encephalopathy and Korsakov's psychosis were two aspects of the same disease. The former was due to acute thiamine deficiency precipitated by intercurrent disease, such as dysentry, exacerbating the effects of a diet lacking the vitamin. The latter was due to a chronically deficient intake such as occurs when malnutrition is due to poor food or, in alcoholics, the substitution of alcohol for food. In their patients exhibiting the bodily symptoms of beriberi — polyneuritis and heart failure — mild mental symptoms of irritability, anxiety and depression could precede the more severe conditions. Their carefully husbanded supplies of vitamins were inadequate to treat all their patients.[18]

In the opening decades of this century, pellagra was well known in the southern states of the USA. It was so widespread that it was thought to be an infectious disease. Its main incidence was among the poor White and Black populations and in institutions. As in the original descriptions in Spain and Italy, it was seen where maize was the staple, almost only, dietary constituent. It was called the disease of the four Ds — dermatitis, diarrhoea, depression and dementia.

In 1914, Dr Joseph Goldberger of the US Public Health Service was assigned to study the problem. He noted that in institutions there were no cases among nurses and attendants and that fresh cases could occur in inmates who had had no outside contact for a year. In an orphanage in Jackson, Mississippi, the highest incidence was in children between 6 and 12 years of age. The younger children received a ration of fresh milk. The older ones received a supplement of fresh meat as farm workers. The incidence dropped when the diet was improved with animal products and legumes. A 12-month survey of the Georgia State Sanatorium showed a recurrence of the condition in half of a control group when they reverted to the previous restricted diet. Influenced by Eijkman's experience, Goldberger had a group of convicts placed on what he had identified as the deficiency diet and symptoms of pellagra developed in five months.[19]

In Britain pellagra has been seen sporadically in institutions — J.C. Howden reported a case from the Royal Mental Hospital at Montrose in 1868 — and among elderly infirm persons living alone and neglecting their diets. In spite of Goldberger's findings, pellagra persisted and in 1940 in the USA there were still 2000 deaths ascribed to it.[20] Although treatment with nicotinic acid was shown to be successful in 1937, research workers in the 1940s showed that it was not its absence from the diet that was the problem. Not only does maize contain nicotinic acid but the vitamin is also synthesised by bacteria in the large intestine. The trouble apparently lay in a toxic analogue of nicotinic acid in maize which created an increased need for the vitamin which can be supplied from tryptophan, a constituent of protein. Hence the improvement which occurred when the diet was supplemented with animal protein.[21]

## Hormone treatment

The ductless (endocrine) glands are those which secrete their products directly into the bloodstream. These secretions are called hormones, a name coined from the Greek word for messenger by Ernest Starling (1876–1926), the physiologist, in 1905. Increasing knowledge of the endocrine glands and the effects of their hormones led to the hope that their malfunctioning would be found to be the basis of mental illness and that hormone therapy would work wonders. No place was found for pituitary and adrenal gland extracts in treatment, although an adreno-genital syndrome of male hirsutism in women with a paranoid psychosis was claimed to be relieved by surgical removal of the adrenal tumour or a hyperplastic adrenal gland. Atrophic and degenerative changes in the testes of male schizophrenic patients suggested the use of male sex hormones and anterior pituitary extract, but no good resulted. Involutional melancholia — that is, severe depression occurring after the menopause — was treated in the 1940s with various female sex hormones on the supposition that the condition was due to diminution of the ovarian secretions. The results of this treatment were much inferior to those obtained with ECT.[22]

The only hormones which were found to be of value were insulin, as described in insulin coma and the modified treatment, and thyroid extract. Thyroxine, the active principle in thyroid extract, was synthesised by Sir Charles Harington (1897–1972) at University College, London, in 1933 but the extract and the dried gland obtained from animals had been used successfully since the later years of the nineteenth century.

Paracelsus and others described the condition of cretinism, a retardation of physical and mental development in children, which is caused by the failure of the thyroid to produce thyroxine because iodine, its chief constituent, is lacking in the diet.

In 1873, Sir William Gull (1816–90) of Guy's Hospital, London, described 'a cretinoid state supervening in adult life in women'.[23] Interest in this and other reports caused the Clinical Society of London to set up in 1883 a Committee on Myxoedema, so called because the observed thickening of tissues in hypothyroid patients was thought to be an accumulation of mucin. The Chairman of the Committee was William Miller Ord (1834–1902), of St Thomas' Hospital, who in 1877 had demonstrated atrophy of the thyroid in the condition. The Committee appointed (Sir) Victor Horseley (1857–1916) to carry out research and a report was published in 1888. In it was stated: 'Delusions – hallucinations occur in nearly half the cases, mainly where the disease is advanced. Insanity as a complication is noted in about the same proportion as delusions and hallucinations. It takes the form of acute or chronic manias, dementia, or melancholia, with a marked predominance of suspicion and self-accusation.'

The successful treatment of a myxodematous patient with thyroid extract was first carried out by George Redmayne Murray (1865–1939), physician to the Royal Victoria Infirmary, Newcastle-upon-Tyne. He noted the suggestion of Horsley that patients should receive a graft of healthy thyroid gland. Instead, he prepared a glycerin extract of sheep's thyroid which was later incorporated in the British Pharmacopoeia of 1898 as 'liquor thyroidei'. He demonstrated the patient in 1891 at a medical meeting and started her on twice-weekly injections. Later the extract was given by mouth and in 1918 in tablet form. In 1920 he reported that the patient had been kept well until her death at the age of 74.[24]

Although there were published reports of mental illness with myxoedema, it was a diagnosis that could be missed, especially in the early mild case. Attention was drawn to it again in 1949 in a classical paper by Richard Asher entitled 'Myxoedematous Madness' in which he described the successful treatment of nine out of ten patients and the partial recovery of two others.[25]

Of course, thyroid extract was tried in schizophrenia — Kraepelin used it with testicular and ovarian extracts in 1922 — but with no success except in a small and rare group of cases. This was a group of patients who had periodic attacks of catatonia — a state of mutism and disordered movement — who were studied for years in the 1930s by Rolf Gjessing (1889–1959), Superintendent of Dikemark Mental Hospital in Norway and an active Resistance worker during the German occupation. He claimed to terminate the catatonia with thyroxine and a low-protein diet.[26]

## References

1. Thomson W.A.R. (1976). *Herbs that Heal*, London: A. & C. Black.
2. Huson P. (1974). *Mastering Herbalism*. London: Sphere.
3. Coats A.M. (1956). *Flowers and their Histories*. London: A. & C. Black.
4. Brownlow M. (1978). *Herbs and the Fragrant Garden*. London: Dartman Longman Todd.
5. Rohde E.S. *The Old English Herbals*.
6. Hunter R.A., Macalpine I. (1963). *Three Hundred Years of Psychiatry 1535–1860*, p. 487. Oxford University Press.
7. Hordern A. (1968). Some historical considerations. In *Psychopharmacology* (Joyce C.R.B., ed.) London: Tavistock.
8. Lader M. The history of psychopharmacology. In *The S.K. & F. History of British Psychiatry*. Welwyn Garden City: Smith, Kline & French Laboratories.
9. Ayd F.J., Blackwell B., eds (1970). *Discoveries in Biological Psychiatry*. Philadelphia: Lippincott.
   — Deniker P. Introduction of neuroleptic therapy,
   — *Ibid*. pp. 155-64.
   — Janssen P.A.J. The butyrophenone story, *Ibid*. pp.165-79.
   — Raven J.F. The history of the thioxanthines, *Ibid*. pp.180-93.
   — Kline N. Monoamine oxidase inhibitors, *Ibid*. pp.194-204
   — Cohen I.M. The benzodiazepines, *Ibid*. pp.130-41.
10. Sim M. (1974). *Guide to Psychiatry*, p. 840. Edinburgh–London: Churchill Livingstone.
11. Kuhn R. (1958). The treatment of depressive states with G22355 (Imipramine Hydrochloride). *American Journal of Psychiatry*; **115**:459.
12. Cade J.F.J. (1949). Lithium salts in the treatment of psychotic excitement. *Medical Journal of Australia*; **1**:195.
13. Baastrup P.C., Schou M. (1967). Lithium as a prophylactic agent. *Archives of General Psychiatry*; **16**:162.
14. Baastrup P.C., Poulsen J.C., Schou M., Thomsen K. (1970). Prophylactic Lithium: double blind discontinuation. *Lancet*; **ii**:326.
15. Major R.H. (1978). *Classic Descriptions of Disease*. Springfield, Ill: Charles C. Thomas.
16. Hunter R.A., Macalpine I. (1963). *Op.cit*. p. 739.
17. De Wardener H.E., Lennox B. (1947). Cerebral beri-beri (Wernicke's encephalopathy). *Lancet*; **ii**:11.
18. Lishman W.A. (1978). *Organic Psychiatry*. Oxford: Blackwell.
19. Cooper B., Morgan H.G. (1973). *Epidemiological Psychiatry*. Springfield, Ill: Charles C. Thomas.
20. Roe D.A. (1973). *A Plague of Corn*. Ithaca and London: Cornell University Press.

21. Hardwick S.W. (1949). Vitamin deficiency in nervous and mental disorder. In *Recent Progress in Psychiatry* Vol. 2 (G.W.T.H. Fleming ed.) p. 115. London: Churchill.

22. Hemphill R.E. (1944). Endocrinology in clinical psychiatry. In *Recent Progress in Psychiatry*. (Fleming G.W.T.H., ed.) p. 417. London: Churchill.

23. Major R.H. (1978). *Op.cit.*, p.268.

24. Murray G.R. (1920). The life history of the first case of myxoedema treated by thyroid extract. *British Medical Journal*; **1**:359.

25. Asher R. (1949). Myxoedematous madness: *Ibid*; **2**:555.

26. Froshaug H., Johannessen N.B. (1958). The seventieth birthday of R. Gjessing. *Journal of Mental Science*; **104**:822.

# II: The Psychotherapies

## CHAPTER 6

# *The Beginnings*

In 1853, Walter Cooper Dendy (1794–1871), a surgeon, read a paper to the Medical Society of London entitled 'Psychotherapeia or the remedial influence of mind'. He defined pyschotherapy as 'prevention and remedy (of disease) by physical influence'. In his paper he said: 'As we know that mental states induce disorder, we may also perceive that prevention and cure may be effected simply by inducing a contrary condition of mind'.[1]

Another definition of psychotherapy is that it comprises all those methods of treatment in which the patient's condition is modified by the thoughts, feelings and non-invasive actions of another person or persons. Psychotherapy can be used alone or can complement or be complemented by physical methods and/or social measures. The range of psychotherapy is wide. At its simplest it is the capacity for empathy with the patient which every good healer has, and it implies his or her awareness of the psychosocial accompaniments of disease. At its most elaborate it is a treatment carried out by a person trained in a special technique based on a rational, coherent theory of mental mechanisms which can be conveyed or interpreted to the patient in a meaningful way through an intense formal relationship.

What all the psychotherapies have in common is a confiding relationship with a helping person and an understanding, which may be dim or clear, of the difference between the outer symptom and the inner experience or cause. The psychotherapeutic techniques aim to get beyond the conscious defence, distortion or rationalisation and reach the subconscious or unconscious reality. The principles were known to the ancients. Centuries before Freud and Jung, the Greek priest-physicians used dream interpretation. In the third century BC, when Antiochus, later named Soter, went into a depressive decline, his father, Seleneus Nicator, King of Syria, summoned Eristratus, a court physician from Egypt. Eristratus noted a rise in the prince's pulse rate at the sight or mention of his young stepmother, Stratonice, and interpreted the illness as an expression of a severe emotional conflict. This was resolved when Seleneus ceded his wife to his son.

## Mesmerism

Most psychotherapeutic techniques are founded on theories of mental mechanisms or organisations. These theories are not to be thought of in the scientific sense as orderly deductions from verifiable observations, but rather as ideas, speculations even, some more rationally coherent and systematised than others. The fact that a psychotherapy helps patients does not prove the soundness of the underlying theory.[2] Mesmerism is an early example. Franz Anton Mesmer (1734–1815) was a graduate of Vienna. Richard Mead (1673–1754), second owner of the famous gold-headed cane, impressed by Newton's discovery of the gravitational attraction between heavenly bodies, wrote a treatise on the influence of the sun and moon on human bodies in producing disease. Mesmer followed him in postulating a cosmic force acting on the nervous system which he called 'animal gravitation' and, when he found that he could get good results by applying magnets to the seats of disease, he conceived the idea that there was in the body a magnetic fluid, the stuff of 'animal magnetism', and that he was restoring its equilibrium and harmonious flow with the application of his magnets and metallic conductors. A country priest, Fr. John Joseph Gassner, was renowned for his cures of nervous complaints and Mesmer noted when he met him that he produced his effects by manipulation alone. This is reminiscent of the stroking treatment of Valentine Greatrakes (1629–83), the Irish ex-soldier, whose claims for cures were attested by the Honourable Robert Boyle, the scientist, among others. Mesmer then discarded the magnets and claimed that the animal magnetism flowed from his body to the bodies of his patients and provoked therapeutic crises in the form of convulsions and other phenomena. His extravagant claims aroused opposition and he moved to Paris in 1779. There he heightened the effects of his hand passes and eye fixations by treating patients in a darkened room

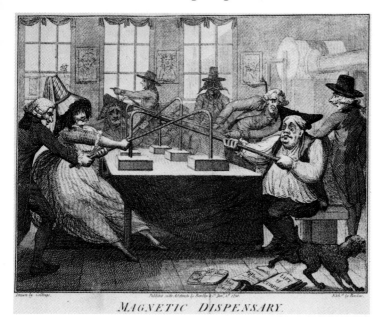

MAGNETIC DISPENSARY

*An eighteenth century psychiatric outpatient clinic*

and with background music. His baquet was a covered tub, for the magnetic fluid, to which the patients were connected by cords or rods. The alarm of the medical faculty resulted in the appointment of a royal commission in 1784, among whose members were Benjamin Franklin, Antoine Lavoisier, the chemist, and Dr Guillotin. They reported that they found no evidence of magnetism and attributed all the observed phenomena to 'the imagination (which) is that active and terrible power'. This drove Mesmer into retirement in Germany and Switzerland where he continued to argue against the psychological nature of the system which his followers were spreading throughout Europe in the first decades of the nineteenth century.[3]

In spite of opposition from those involved in orthodox medicine, mesmerism continued to be used by non-medical practitioners. It received a great fillip in England when John Elliotson (1791–1868), the brilliant but unconventional Professor of Medicine at University College Hospital, London, espoused its cause in 1837. Controversy caused Elliotson's resignation from his Chair in 1838 but he continued to practise mesmerism in parallel with a consulting medical practice.[4] He did not force his mesmeric methods on patients who did not opt for them. Another who brought mesmerism into prominence was James Esdaile (1808–1859), a surgeon in India, who, before chemical anaesthesia was established, was operating on mesmerised patients. In 1845, having had success in soothing a patient after operation with 'mesmeric passes', a week later he performed a second operation after rendering him unconscious and analgesic. His *Mesmerism in India, and its practical application in surgery and medicine* (1846) enhanced his reputation and led to his appointment by the Governor-General in 1848 to the post of Residency Surgeon.[4] When the American Congress in 1853 offered $100 000 to the true discoverer of the anaesthetic properties of ether, he addressed to them an indignant protest denying that ether had preceded mesmerism.

## Hypnotism

This is the term, shortened from neuro-hypnotism, which was coined by James Braid (1795–1860), a Scottish doctor who practised in Manchester. A lecture there by the French mesmerist, La Fontaine, in 1841 interested Braid in animal magnetism. His researches showed him that the mesmeric trance could be self-induced by the subject's concentration and fixation on an inanimate object. This drew on him the wrath of the mesmerists, upset by his devaluation of the virtue and influence of the operator. He countered their arguments calmly and also published his critical views on magic, witchcraft, table-moving and spirit-rapping. Braid's hypnotism was introduced into France when Dr Azam wrote an article about it in 1859 in the *Archives de Médécine*. Dr Broca, famous as a neuroanatomist, spoke about it to the Académie des Sciences in the following year, and it was in France that hypnotism made its greatest advances.[4,8]

Auguste Ambrose Liébeault (1823–1904) set up in general medical practice in Nancy in 1864. He had been interested in mesmerism for some years and used hypnotic sleep for treatment and research. He became popular not only because of his cures but because he did not charge those patients who elected to have hypnotism. Hippolyte Bernheim (1837–1919), Professor of Neurology at Nancy, visited Liébeault in 1880 because he had cured a patient whom Bernheim had diagnosed as having sciatica. He was very impressed with Liébeault's methods and accepted his views on the influence of the

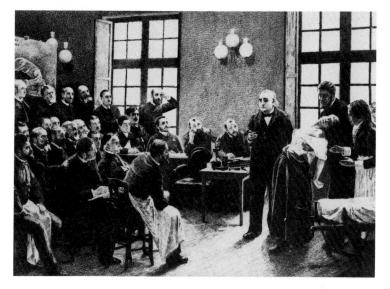

*Charcot lecturing on hysteria at the Salpêtrière. J. F. Babinski is the man supporting the patient, Pierre Marie is the third man seated on Charcot's right. This picture, by André Brouillet, hung in Freud's consulting room in Vienna and later in London*

mental on the physical. He went on to collect a series of 5000 cases in four years and in 1886 published a book on suggestion and its therapeutic applications.[5]

While Bernheim was building up an impressive collection of clinical experience at Nancy, there was at the Salpêtrière in Paris a rival school. Jean Martin Charcot (1825–93) was physician and neurologist there and became interested in hypnosis (to use the modern term) in 1878. Patients with functional nervous illness — that is, those with symptoms and signs such as paralysis or tremor or weakness or local abnormal sensation without evidence of structural or organic change in the nervous system — were referred to physicians, particularly neurologists, and surgeons. Sir Benjamin Brodie (1783–1862), the eminent surgeon to whom the first edition of *Gray's Anatomy* was dedicated, published a book of *Lectures illustrative of certain local nervous affections* in which he displayed notable psychological insight when he wrote that 'fear, suggestion and unconscious simulation are the primary factors'.[4] It was only the obviously deranged who were dealt with by psychiatrists or alienists. Hysteria was the favoured diagnosis for this group of disorders. What Sir Charles Bell (1774–1842) said of William Cullen's (1710–90) systematic classification of diseases, which included the neuroses, applies very much to hysteria: 'nominal varieties are made diseases when there is no real distinction'. Because there was a name, hysteria was presumed to have an identity. (The identity of hysteria was still being proposed and opposed in the 1960s).

As a neurologist, Charcot had many hysterical patients referred to him and these were the subject of his investigation of hypnosis. The responses of patients to his thorough neurological investigations of their paralyses and anaesthesias convinced Charcot that these characteristic states could only be produced in persons who suffered from hysteria and that he could draw up an impressive list of the stigmata of the disorder. Bernheim pointed out that all these phenomena were the products of suggestion and that suggestibility was not limited to hysterical patients. Indeed, Liébeault told an English visitor, Dr J.M. Bramwell, that the nervous and hysterical were his most refractory subjects.[6]

Charcot was a brilliant showman as well as a first-class physician and his demonstrations of his three stages of hypnotic sleep — lethargy, catalepsy and somnambulism — were famous throughout Europe. A vivid description of the atmosphere of the Salpêtrière is given by Axel Munthe in his autobiography *The Story of San Michele*. Among the visitors to Charcot's clinic was Sigmund Freud (1856–1939) who went there while holding a travelling scholarship in 1885. Later Freud paid tribute to Charcot's valuable clinical descriptions while pointing out that he treated the problems of the neuroses from the standpoint of the pathological anatomy in which he had been trained and showed no interest in their psychology. The man who did draw psychological conclusions from the work at the Salpêtrière was Pierre Janet (1859–1947). From his studies of hysterics, he derived the concept of dissociation: 'Things happen as if an idea, a partial system of thoughts, emancipated itself and developed on its own account'.[7] Other concepts of his resembled the 'unconscious' of Freud and his mechanism of repression and catharsis, the complex as defined by Jung and the organ inferiority of Adler. However, none of these authorities gave him any great credit for originality. Their criticism of his not having pursued his ideas far enough implies, in each case, that if he had he would have reached the truth as perceived by them. His system of psychotherapy, which he called psychological analysis, did not attract the fame which the others achieved.

It was inevitable that hypnosis would be tried in the treatment of the psychoses. Bramwell and Axel Munthe have both described how Professor Voisin of the Asile St Anne in Paris would try for hours to hypnotise patients struggling in their straitjackets until he gave up or the patient was exhausted. Braid's demonstrations that hypnosis is virtually auto-hypnosis had not been appreciated.

It is customary for writers of textbooks to state that the nature of hypnosis is not yet understood. Nevertheless, certain explanatory statements can be made. There are individuals who communicate easily with others and who have persuasive and suggestive powers. The patient comes to the healer more or less prepared to accept his opinion and ministrations. The technique of hypnosis is some method of inducing the subject to withdraw his awareness from the here and now and to concentrate his attention on the particular portion of his mental content which the hypnotist specifies. Thus, for example, Janet's dissociated material can be identified, understood and reintegrated within the mind. Or faulty reactions to situations can be clarified for the patient, and he can be persuaded to correct inappropriate responses if the original reason for them can be brought into full consciousness. The revival by hypnosis of buried memories of horrifying experiences was used to good effect in the cases of so-called 'shell-shock' in the First World War.

## Psychoanalysis

No system other than the theory and practice originated by Sigmund Freud should be called psychoanalysis. The acceptance of this rigorous definition was due to the efforts of Ernest Jones.

After studying with Charcot, Freud returned to Vienna and commenced private practice in 1886, using hypnosis although he found induction rather arduous. Josef Breuer (1842–1925) was a general practitioner who was treating neurotic patients by getting them to talk freely under hypnosis. After Freud had visited Liébeault and Bernheim at Nancy in 1889, he realised the possibility of unconscious mental processes and used Breuer's method of getting the patients to unburden themselves not only of the disturbing memories or fantasies but also of the accompanying emotions. This was catharsis or purging of the mind. He and Breuer published a paper in 1893 and a book, *Studies in Hysteria*, in 1895. Then Freud found that hypnosis was not necessary when a patient, Elizabeth, obviously a forthright young lady, complained of his interruptions while she was in full flow. He therefore got the patients to talk in full consciousness, urging them not to pick and choose or censor their output. This was free association and the process of analysing and interpreting the patient's productions was psychoanlysis. The classic method with the patient lying on the couch and the analyst sitting behind the patient's range of vision has been made familiar in cartoon and film.

As his practice flourished, Freud found more and more that the repressed and painful memories of his patients related to traumatic sexual experiences in childhood: seduction or the witnessing of parental intercourse. Breuer could not accept the sexual causation of the neuroses and he, the first of Freud's collaborators or disciples, was the first to part company with him. Further study of the unconscious mental processes led Freud to an interest in dreams and in 1900 he published *The Interpretation of Dreams*. In 1904, *The Psychopathology of Everyday Life*, a study of errors and lapses of memory and slips of the tongue, appeared and, in 1905, *Three Contributions to the Theory of Sex* introduced, among other things, new ideas in child psychology.

In 1903 he founded The Psychological Wednesday Society, from which was formed, in 1908, the Vienna Psychoanalytic Society. The first International Congress of Psychoanalysis was held at Salzburg in 1908 and in 1909 the International Psychoanalytical Association was formed to set standards for psychoanalysis and regulate the practice of psychoanalysis by approved practitioners. Freud's *Introductory Lectures on Psychoanalysis* were given at Clark University in 1909 and spread his ideas in the USA. He continued to treat patients, refine and elaborate his ideas, write books on psychoanlaysis and psychoanalytical studies of subjects in literature and art and history, and keep up a voluminous correspondence until his death in 1939. His work with patients was interrupted several times by treatment for a recurrent cancer of the mouth — he was a heavy and persistent smoker of cigars — and finally in 1938 when his friends eventually persuaded him to leave Nazi-dominated Vienna for London.[9]

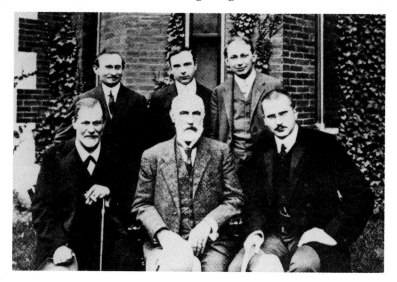

Group: *Worcester, Massachusetts, September 1909*
*A. A. Brill, Ernest Jones, Sandor Ferenczi,*
*Freud, Stanley Hall, C. G. Jung*

## Analytical psychology

Burghölzli was the cantonal mental hospital for Zurich and housed the Psychiatric Department of the University. Eugen Bleuler (1857–1939) was Professor there from 1898, and in 1900 Carl Gustav Jung (1875–1961) joined him as one of his assistants. Bleuler and his assistants became interested in psychoanalysis in 1906 and attended the Congress in Salzburg in 1908. Two others from Burghölzli who became well known psychoanalysts were Karl Abraham and A.A. Brill, who translated Freud's early works for the benefit of the English-speaking world and who was one of the founders of the American Psychoanalytic Association in 1911.

Freud was much encouraged by the support of the academic and hospital-based psychiatrists and proposed, at the second Congress held in Nuremburg in 1910, that Jung should be Life-President of their International Association.

His Viennese adherents Stekel and Adler violently opposed this but, after an impassioned plea by Freud that an official psychiatrist and Gentile should head the movement, they agreed to Jung's election for a two-year term.

It was not long before Jung started to diverge from Freud's teaching. He rejected the primacy of the sexual instinct. For him, libido
was a life force. The unconscious mind did contain some repressed
material as Freud taught, but Jung placed most emphasis on the
collective unconscious which contained the myths and beliefs of the
race to which the individual belonged. The break with the
Psychoanalysts came in 1913 and Jung went on to develop his
analytical psychology.

Introvert, extravert and complex are psychological terms not
invented by Jung but given by him a wider currency. Archetypes
were the symbols of universal concepts, products of the collective
unconscious, which he found in his analyses and which he used in
interpreting neuroses. Like Freud, he used dream material. His later
work on psychological types, reminiscent of Galen's four temperaments, was well received by psychiatrists who were not his followers. Jung said that his theory of types was founded on his observations of Freud, Adler and himself during the early dissensions, and he
also suggested that there were patients who were best treated on
Freudian lines, others on Adlerian lines and others according to his
own method.[10]

## Individual psychology

Alfred Adler was one of the Wednesday evening discussion circle
which started meeting at Freud's house in 1902. He had set up in
private practice in 1898, showed an interest in the social aspects and
then the psychological aspects of illness and had been influenced by
the ideas of Janet. One version of his first connection with Freud is
that he defended his views after a lecture which the Viennese doctors
had received with hostility.

In 1907 he published his monograph on the *Inferiority of Organs*, in
which he based the origin of the neuroses on the mental influence of
physical deficits. After the turmoil of the 1910 Congress, Adler tried
to adapt his theory to Freud's and Freud invited him to lecture on his
research. In three lectures early in 1911 he set out his criticism of the
sexual theory and his own idea of the masculine protest. At three
sessions of discussion which followed, the Freudian adepts (the term
used by Franz Wittels) made what looked like a concerted attack on
Adler's ideas. At the final session Stekel attempted a reconciliation
but it was Freud himself who pointed out the impossibility of

agreement. This led to Adler's resignation as President of the Vienna Psychoanalytic Society and, with the publication in 1912 of his book, *The Neurotic Constitution*, which incorporated what he had learned from Janet on neurosis and from Freud on mental mechanisms, he had founded his 'individual psychology'. Eight members who seceded from the Society with Adler comprised a professor of education, two philosophers, a speech therapist and four doctors.

Adler's rejection of the sexual theory, his ideas that strivings could be compensations for deficits and that neuroses could be the expression of an inferiority complex, appeared nearer to common sense and everyday experience than Freud's ideas and appealed to non-medical thinkers.

During the First World War, Adler treated psychiatric casualties. After the War he became interested in the problems of homeless and delinquent children, helped to establish child guidance clinics in Vienna and lectured to teachers and parents on child development and education. The first International Congress of Individual Psychology took place in Vienna in 1924. His last 15 years were spent in lecturing in Europe and the USA and in treating private patients.[12]

# References

1. Hunter R.A., Macalpine I. (1963). *Three Hundred Years of Psychiatry 1535–1860*, p. 1004. Oxford: Oxford University Press.
2. Popper K. (1953). Science: conjectures and refutations. In *British Philosophy in Mid-century* (Mace C.A., ed.) pp.33–9. London: Routledge and Kegan Paul.
3. Buranelli V. (1975). *The Wizard from Vienna*. New York: Coward, McCann.
4. Hunter R.A., Macalpine I. (1963). *Op.cit.* pp.482, 860, 906.
5. Zilboorg G. (1941). *A History of Medical Psychology*. New York: Norton.
6. Bramwell J.M. (1930). *Hypnotism, its History, Practice and Theory*. Philadelphia: Lippincott.
7. Janet P. (1906). *The Major Symptoms of Hysteria*. New York: Macmillan.
8. Reeves J.W. (1958). *Body and Mind in Western Thought*. Harmondsworth: Penguin.
9. Clark R.W. (1980). *Freud: The Man and the Cause*. London: Jonathan Cape.
10. Fordham F. (1956). *An Introduction to Jung's Psychology*. Harmondsworth: Penguin.
11. Wittels F. (1924). *Sigmund Freud, His Personality, His Teachings and His School*. London: Allen & Unwin.
12. Way L. (1956). *Alfred Adler: An Introduction to his Psychology*. Harmondsworth: Penguin.

# CHAPTER 7

# The Expansion of Psychotherapy

## The later history of psychoanalysis

After the schisms of Adler and Jung, Ernest Jones (1879–1958), Freud's first British follower and his biographer, formed a committee of senior analysts pledged to uphold the basic Freudian concepts. It consisted of Ferenczi, Abraham, Eitingon, Rank, Sachs and himself. He founded the British Psychoanalytic Society in 1919. Karl Abraham (1877–1925), who had been at Burgholzli with Bleuler and Jung, was one of the founders of the Berlin Psychoanalytic Institute in 1920, and the Institutes in New York and Chicago started in 1931 and 1932 respectively. They were centres of training and of treatment because it had been agreed that recognition as psychoanalysts could only be given to those who had been through a period of study, personal analysis and supervised therapy.

In a movement of highly intelligent individuals, engaged in novel and emotionally charged practices, there were bound to be dissensions and theoretical differences. An analysis by the Freudian method of free association, acceptance and resolution of blocks and resistances, painstaking pursuit of all subjects brought up by the patient and repeated interpretations, was a long and expensive process which could last two or three or more years. Efforts to shorten the treatment were frowned on by Freud. This led to a parting with Wilhelm Stekel (1868–1940) who instituted active therapy, stimulating the production of unconscious material by imposing restrictions in the patient's life.

Sandor Ferenczi (1873–1933), who did not wish to break with Freud but was disowned by him in 1932, had transgressed by abandoning the analyst's uninvolved attitude and entering into an encouraging and approving relationship with the patient. Otto Rank (1884–1939) left the orthodox group in 1934. He had imposed a time limit on treatment, and his theory that the trauma of birth was more important than infantile sexuality could not be tolerated.

Karen Horney (1885–1952) and Erich Fromm (b. 1900) were analysts at the Berlin Institute for 15 years. In the early 1930s they moved to the USA while Anna Freud and Melanie Klein moved to England. The Nazis caused an injection of continental psychiatry into the English-speaking world. Horney and Fromm together with Harry Stack Sullivan (1892–1948) became known as the neo-Freudian school of analysts. Anna Freud and Melanie Klein worked with children. They differed in technique: Anna Freud pursued verbal methods with children from the age of 3 years; Melanie Klein used a free association play therapy with even younger patients. There were inevitably differences in their teachings on the development of the child. Ernest Jones supported the Kleinian view rather than that of his mentor's daughter.[1]

## Psychotherapy progresses

The large number of psychiatric casualties in the First World War proved to be an impetus to the development of psychotherapy methods. The neurological view of 'shell shock' and 'concussion' did not lead to successful treatment but the depth psychology derived from Freud began to prove helpful. Freud did not treat any soldiers, but in 1920 a commission of investigation asked for his views on Wagner-Jauregg's treatment of neurotic soldiers, which had been the subject of serious complaint.

Adler was head of a hospital for psychiatric casualties in Vienna. David Eder in Berlin found six patients suitable for psychoanalysis among 100 cases of war neurosis. Babinski and Froment, formerly with Charcot, worked with French soldiers. In Britain (Sir) Arthur Hurst (1879–1944), a physician of Guy's Hospital, treated war neurosis at Netley Military Hospital and at Seale Hayne. He favoured counter-suggestion. William McDougall (1871–1938) with experience in medicine, neurology and anthropology, used hypnoanalysis in treating casualties. He was assisted at Oxford by J.A. Hadfield. W.H.R. Rivers (1864–1922), whose experience was also in neurology and anthropology, worked at the military hospitals at

Maghull and Craiglockhart. He was the psychiatrist described in Siegfried Sassoon's *Complete Memoirs of George Sherston*.

Experience and interest in psychotherapy carried over into civilian life. In 1920, Dr H. Crichton Miller, assisted by J. A. Hadfield and Ian Suttie, founded the Tavistock Clinic which has continued to be a centre of teaching, research and therapy ever since.[2] Among the distinguished members of its staff may be mentioned John Bowlby and his work on maternal separation; Wilfred Bion who was a pioneer in group therapy; and H.V. Dicks who did illuminating work in marital problems. In the early 1950s Michael Balint, a pupil of Ferenczi, instituted a widely copied series of seminars with general practitioners. Brief psychotherapy has been taught from the Tavistock by David Malan.

Also in 1920 was founded the Cassel Hospital, now at Richmond, Surrey.[2] It was one of the last benefactions of Sir Ernest Cassel (1852–1921), financier and philanthropist and grandfather of Edwina, Countess Mountbatten. Dr T.A. Ross, Medical Director until 1934, practised a shorter form of psychotherapy based on the explanation, persuasion and suggestion methods of Dubois and Dejerine. His book, *The Common Neuroses*, introduced psychotherapy to a wider audience of doctors. After the Second World War, Dr T.F. Main broadened the hospital's scope. Psychotherapy was psychoanalytic in nature and special work has been done in puerperal mental illness, family therapy and the formation of a therapeutic community.

In family therapy the presenting patient is not treated in isolation. He or she is seen as a member of a family group and the other members are invited to join in the therapeutic process. This has been practised and taught also at the Institute of Family Therapy in Ipswich since 1957.

Psychotherapy has not been a conspicuously successful treatment of the psychoses. Ferenczi attempted it in Budapest. In 1946 and 1947, J.N. Rosen reported some success in lengthy sessions — up to 16 hours — with schizophrenic patients in which he accepted the reality of the patient's psychotic world, but there was no stampede to follow him.[3]

## Psychotherapy in the Second World War

The appointment of Dr J.R. Rees from the Tavistock Clinic as Director of Army Psychiatry ensured that psychotherapy would not be overlooked. The practical implications of Wilhelm Stekel's active therapy had appealed to therapists who did not wholeheartedly subscribe to psychoanalysis, and there were various adaptations.

From 1931, J.S. Horsley had been using intravenous barbiturates to effect a quicker mobilisation of unconscious material and this method was used by William Sargant and Eliot Slater to treat casualties from Dunkirk and the London blitz at Belmont Hospital. Horsley called his method narcoanalysis.[4] R.R. Grinker and J.P. Spiegel, who used it in an American military hospital in North Africa, called it narcosynthesis.[5] H.A. Palmer in the Western Desert campaign (1942–3) used the excitatory effect of inhaled ether to produce an abreaction of repressed traumatic memories and anxiety.[6] This was also used in the UK by Sargant and Shorvon.[7] Chloroform and ether had also been given for this purpose in the First World War, and before that John Snow in 1858 had used chloroform in the relief of hysterical paralysis.

Mild cases of psychoneurosis occurring in Service personnel were treated by superficial psychotherapy consisting of an adequate personal history, explanation and reassurance and the avoidance of analytical technique.

Nevertheless, it was pointed out that the Freudian transference situation was being used by the medical officer as father-figure and that treating the patients in small groups did not necessarily evade it. Anxious and hypersensitive patients were desensitised to air-raid noises by listening to gramophone records of sirens, AA gunfire and explosions. The method could be used to produce abreaction. After exposure to the sounds, pulse and respiration rates were recorded and with repetition the diminished responses were shown to the patients and combined with explanation and reassurance.

Effort syndrome (as Da Costa's syndrome, it was described in the American Civil War) is a neurosis with fears of heart disease suggested by the palpitations induced by anxiety. In the early years of the Second World War it was so common that a special treatment unit was set up at Mill Hill EMS Hospital. There, Maxwell Jones gave lectures on the structure and function of the nervous system and the true significance of the symptoms. This had little effect. Improvement was obtained when the emotional attitude of the patients was examined with them and they were able to discuss their feelings with nurses, who appreciated the psychological mechanisms.[8]

In the later years of the War, neurotic patients were beginning to accumulate in military hospitals faster than they could be dealt with. Overseas commands with limited accommodation were invaliding to the UK patients who needed prolonged treatment, and delays in repatriation had an adverse effect. At Northfield Military Hospital, W.R. Bion and J. Rickman tackled the problem by initiating group psychotherapy. This was more profound than the group provision of explanation and suggestion — the didactic groups. The psychiatrist would be in the group but not its leader. The psychological material was provided by the members, who would not be so numerous as to exclude the less assertive from taking part, and the psychiatrist had to provide interpretations without being overbearing.[9] The later history of those groups was described by S.H. Foulkes in 1948.[10]

This work was carried back to the Tavistock Clinic in peacetime and some form of group psychotherapy has become available in most psychiatric clinics since then.

## The therapeutic community

The dynamics perceived in group psychotherapy led therapists to the concept of the therapeutic community. The term is credited to T.F. Main who, in 1946 with his former colleagues, described the advances made at Northfield Military Hospital, Birmingham.[11] Their experience of a non-directive role converted them into advocating 'a therapeutic setting with a spontaneous and emotionally structured (rather than a medically dictated) organisation in which all staff and patients engaged'. The characteristics of such an organisation have been described as permissiveness — the tolerance of disturbed behaviour; reality confrontation — other members making individuals face up to the results and the meaning of their behaviour; equality — the abolition of marks of difference between patients and staff, such as uniforms, and the use of Christian names; and democracy — participation of all members of the community in decision making, even questions of admission and discharge. The ideas were put into practice in various settings. Main took them to the Cassel Hospital, as already mentioned. Maxwell Jones opened an Industrial Neurosis Unit at Belmont Hospital in 1946 for those unable to work. It became the Social Rehabilitation Unit, and in 1959 the Henderson Hospital. Since then it has been distinguished for accepting the severely maladjusted who have failed elsewhere. Maxwell Jones left there in 1959 and worked in Salem Hospital, Oregon. From 1963 to 1970, he employed his methods at Dingleton Hospital, Melrose, which George Bell had made into the first fully open mental hospital in Britain in 1959. After 1970 he returned to the USA to work at Fort Logan.

D.V.Martin developed a therapeutic community at Claybury Hospital[12] and D.H. Clark did similarly at Fulbourn Hospital, Cambridge.[13] Other therapeutic communities were established as units in larger mental hospitals and in the psychiatric units of general hospitals. The principles of communal treatment were applied in in-patient clinics for the treatment of alcoholism and drug addiction and for adolescent disorders. Outside the hospital setting, some residential units for the resettlement of discharged patients, such as the Richmond Fellowship, were organised on therapeutic community lines and so was Grendon Underwood which the Prison Commissioners staffed with psychiatrically trained medical and prison officers.

Villa 21 at Shenley Hospital started as a therapeutic community for young schizophrenic patients and then gave up the ward meetings and feedback of experience which characterise the therapeutic community in favour of a family approach.[14]

The enthusiasm for group psychotherapy and the therapeutic community could, for some patients, be carried too far. A patient writing in *The Lancet* in 1965 described his despair at his failure to improve in such a setting and his recovery in a conventional unit with drug treatment,[15] and one of the practitioners of community therapy in a review observes 'Yet it is the very cult-like nature of the therapeutic community which can be its undoing, raising expectations and hampering the independence and difference which it aims to tolerate'.[16]

## Action techniques in psychotherapy

Freud's free association and interpetation and the analysis of the transference between patients and therapist are verbal methods. There are, of course, other ways in which emotion and unconscious material can be expressed. Action techniques employ movement, mime, acting, simulation, tactile sensation, non-verbal auditory activity and play to bring out hidden conflicts and suggest solutions.

In Ancient Greece the therapeutic value of drama was recognised. Family conflicts and madness were frequently portrayed and Aristotle put forward the idea that one of the functions of the drama was catharsis, the purging of the emotions. Music, dancing, poetic rhythms and the chanting of the chorus heightened the effect. The most impressive surviving part of the healing temple at Epidaurus is the theatre.

Psychodrama was developed by Jacob Levy Moreno (1892–1974), a Rumanian who set up the Theatre of Spontaneity (Stegreiftheater) in Vienna in 1921. He describes how he used a series of roles and situations to relieve the marital discord of two of his players. When he moved to the USA in 1925, he elaborated his method using a protagonist, i.e. the patient, with a director or therapist, auxiliary egos representing the people in the patient's life and a group which could, like the Greek chorus, provide a commentary or try out an alternative interpretation. In some instances the protagonist was hypnotised on the stage to reduce inhibition.[17]

At Belmont, Maxwell Jones used rehearsed psychodrama. The patient would write or be helped to write a playlet portraying one or more significant incidents in his life. Catharsis and revelation could come during the rehearsal. Didactic psychodrama involved members of the staff playing the parts of the patient and his relatives to make an interpretation acceptable to the patient. The technique of the empty chair is to address the fantasised person sitting in it. The patient is not interacting with the group but performing before it.

Fritz Perls (1894–1970) devised Gestalt therapy in which the patient has to personify the warring parts of his body or mind and invent a dialogue in which they could come to agreement, completing the gestalt (or wholeness).

In therapeutic games, the members of a group are encouraged to shed inhibitions, but not pressed to join in, and try to express and experience feelings in active or symbolic ways: dancing, singing, shouting of slogans, touching others, gently exploring another's face, wrestling, expressing the idea of growth or joy or horror, imitating a train, acting a nursery rhyme, joining in a singing game, etc. With some patients these activities may arouse anxiety or aggression and the therapist must be skilled enough to recognise the possibilities and direct the action into less disturbing channels.[18] The ideas of using posture and body contact had their origin in the writings on body language of Wilhelm Reich (1897–1957), with

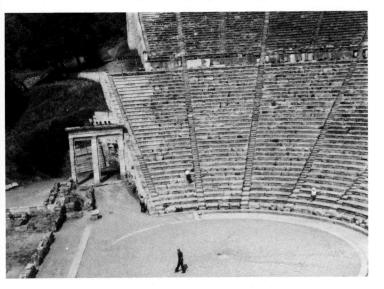

*The theatre at Epidaurus*

whom Perls studied and who began as an orthodox psychoanalyst and deviated when he rejected Freud's death instinct in 1933.

Ronald Laing, in developing his ideas on the causes and treatment of schizophrenia in 1965, had a special 'rumpus room' at Gartnavel for regressed psychotic patients.

T-groups developed in the late 1940s from the ideas of Kurt Lewin, a social psychologist. Transactions between members consisted of self-disclosure with complete honesty and consequent mutual interpretation. They were advocated for people who were not ill as a means of education and improvement. They recall Frank Buchman's Oxford Groups of the 1930s. Encounter groups started with Carl Rogers's work in the 1950s. An atmosphere of trust and belief in inherent goodness was the bond between therapist and subject. From experience, it became clear that, as with the games, these techniques were not suitable for everybody and that the therapist had to be able and prepared to handle the anxiety when it was aroused.

## Meditation

As a religious exercise, meditation has been known for more than 2000 years. In essence it is the focusing of attention on a sound, the mantra, or on a significant object or subject. The turning of attention inwards and neglect of external stimuli has sufficient resemblance to hypnosis to warrant its being thought of as a form of autohypnosis.

In the 1950s research on the psychophysiological accompaniments of meditation was done with the co-operation of accomplished yogis in India and Zen adepts in Japan. Later studies in the next two decades confirmed that there are changes in brain activity as indicated on the electro-encephalograph (EEG), reductions in heart and respiration rates and oxygen consumption and in electrical conductance in the skin.[19] The last-named feature has also been found to occur when anxiety is relieved by treatment.

Interest in meditation as a treatment increased in the 1970s when individuals practising transcendental meditation — the standardised form of mantra meditation taught in the West — stopped or reduced their intake of drugs. Trials of the technique have been carried out for the treatment of neurosis and in stress-related conditions such as insomnia, hypertension and migraine. Meditation as a measure to produce relaxation and relief of the bodily symptoms of anxiety in the context of a psychotherapy programme has obvious value. As a self-administered therapy, it should not be expected to produce outstanding results in those conditions which are serious enough to attract medical attention.

## Music therapy

Music is universally recognised to have an effect on the emotions and on behaviour. Foot-tapping tunes, military marches, soothing lullabies and pop rave-ups are obvious examples. As disordered emotions are prominent in mental illness, it is not surprising that music has been used in treatment. In mythology, Apollo of the golden locks is the god of prophecy, of music and of healing.

In Biblical times David played to Saul to bring him out of his melancholy. Bartholomaeus Anglicus in his *De Proprietatibus Rerum*, a thirteenth-century encyclopaedia, wrote of mental patients: 'Let them be gladded with music and some deal occupied'.

Concerts for patients were a feature of the mental hospitals of the Moslem World in the eleventh and twelfth centuries, and at Edirne in the fifteenth century the Sultan Bayazid II appointed three singers, accompanied by flute, violin, flageolet, cymbalom, and lute, who performed on three days per week. At the mental hospital at Manisa, built in 1539, the patients were soothed by the splashing of the fountains and the music of the court orchestra.[20]

Robert Burton (1577–1640) declared in *The Anatomy of Melancholy*, 'Musick is a roaring-meg against melancholy, to rear and revive the languishing soul; affecting not only the ears but the very arteries, the vital and animal spirits, it erects the mind and makes it nimble'.

Dr Johnson's doctor, Richard Brocklesby (1722–97), wrote a book on the application of music to the cure of diseases, and Sir Henry Halford (1766–1844), who was George III's physician, observed the sedative effect of music on the King.[21]

Pinel's pupil Jean Etienne Dominique Esquirol (1772–1840) said that he had often employed music but had rarely been successful with it; he recommended it as an adjunct to other treatment, and experience has shown that that is as much as can be expected of it.[21]

Sir Frederick Mott, the neuropathologist and moving spirit of the Maudsley Hospital, was a man of many interests. He was President of the Society of English Singers and he wrote a book entitled *War Neurosis and Shell Shock*. He concerned himself with the rehabilitation of disabled soldiers, using music for re-education and therapy.[22]

Music in the form of sing-songs, singing games and percussion bands has been used also in mental hospitals for the stimulation of psychogeriatric patients and withdrawn chronic patients. Indeed, some of the earliest compositions of Sir Edward Elgar (1857–1934) were written for the entertainment of the patients at Worcester County Asylum, where he was bandmaster, and were played at the dances there. In the music therapy programme at Horton Hospital, Epsom, which started in 1955, this was found to be just as important as the encouragement of individual performers and ensembles and the choir.[23] It has also been used as a focus for group therapy. Two doctors at Warlingham Park Hospital found that classical music tended to leave members bored or indifferent. The romantic music of Tchaikovsky and Schubert and Chopin produced emotional release. Folk songs improved group cohesion and harmony and enthusiasm.[24] The audience reaction at another hospital was similar when the Council for Music in Hospitals arranged recitals by individual artistes.[25]

Some years ago, the Editor of *World Medicine* conducted a poll among his friends and acquaintances on the use of music as an anti-depressant. Of 74 people, 34 relied on Mozart and 27 on Wagner. Other composers featured were Bach (19), Beethoven (18), Verdi (14), Scarlatti (8), Ravel (7), Debussy (6), Mahler (6), Johann Strauss (5), Tchaikovsky (4), Delius (1) and Bruch (1). The only non-classical composer to be mentioned was Noel Coward (1) but it would have been interesting to know of others. Medication for depression had also been received by 33 people, 27 of whom claimed that music was more effective.[26]

# References

1. Brown J.A.C. (1964). *Freud and the Post-Freudians*. Harmondsworth: Penguin.
2. Editorial. (1980). *British Medical Journal*; 26th July.
3. Rosen J.N. (1953). *Direct Analysis*. New York: Grune & Stratton.
4. Horsley J.S. (1931). *Narcoanalysis*. London: Oxford University Press.
5. Grinker R.R., Spiegel J.P. (1945). *Men Under Stress*. Philadelphia: Blakiston.
6. Palmer H.A. (1945). *Abreactive techniques — ether. Journal of the Royal Army Medical Corps*; **84**:86.
7. Sargant W. (1967). *The Unquiet Mind* p. 107. London: Heinemann.
8. Crichton Miller H., Nicolle G.H. (1949). Psychotherapy. In *Recent Progress in Psychiatry*, Vol. 2 (Fleming G.W.T.H., ed.) p.307 London: Churchill.
9. Bion W.R., Rickman J. (1943). *Lancet*, **ii**:678.
10. Foulkes S.H. (1948). *An Introduction to Group Analytical Psychotherapy* London: Heinemann.
11. Main T.F. (1946). The hospital as a therapeutic institution. *Bulletin of the Menninger Clinic*, **10**:66.
12. Martin D.V. (1962). *Adventure in Psychiatry*. London: Cassirer.
13. Clark D.H. (1974). *Social Therapy in Psychiatry*. Harmondsworth: Penguin.
14. Laing R.D., Cooper D., Esterson A. (1965). Results of family-orientated therapy in hospitalised schizophrenics. *British Medical Journal*; **2**:1462.
15. Cox J. (1965). A patient's view of psychotherapy *Lancet*; **ii**:678.
16. Mandelbrote B. (1979). Reading about the therapeutic community. *British Journal of Psychiatry*; **135**:369.
17. Moreno J.L. (1959). Psychodrama. In *American Handbook of Psychiatry* (Arieti S., ed.) pp.1375-96. New York: Basic Books.
18. Aveline M. (1979). Action techniques in psychotherapy. *British Journal of Hospital Medicine*; **22/1**:78.
19. West M. (1979). Meditation. *British Journal of Psychiatry*; **135**:457.

20. Volkan V.D. (1975). Turkey. In *World History of Psychiatry* (Howells J.G., ed.) pp.383–99. London: Baillière Tindall.
21. Hunter R.A., Macalpine I. (1963). *Three Hundred Years of Psychiatry 1535*–1860, pp. 376, 377. Oxford: Oxford University Press.
22. Meyer A. (1973). Frederick Mott, Founder of the Maudsley Laboratories. *British Journal of Psychiatry*; **122**:497.
23. Rollin H.R. (1973). The History of Music Therapy. *History of Medicine*; **5**:15.
24. Mitchell S.D., Zanker A. (1948). The use of music in group therapy. *Journal of Mental Science*; **94**:737.
25. Author's observation.
26. O'Donnell M. (1974). Editorial. *World Medicine*; 4th December.

# CHAPTER 8

# *Behaviour Therapy*

Psychoanalysis started from the consulting room. Behaviour therapy came from the psychology laboratory. In 1875, Wilhelm Wundt (1832–1920) founded the first psychology laboratory at Leipzig. His student, G. Stanley Hall (1844–1924), opened the first in the USA at Johns Hopkins University in 1881. It was he who, as President of Clark University, invited Freud to give the introductory lectures on psychoanalysis in 1909.

John Broadus Watson (1878–1958) became Professor of Psychology at Johns Hopkins University in 1908. There he continued the work on learning in laboratory animals which he had been doing in the University of Chicago. In 1913 he published a paper in which he claimed that the objective methods used to study animal behaviour were the only useful ones in the study of human behaviour, psychology was essentially the study of behaviour, and 'consciousness', 'mind', 'mental state' and 'imagination' could not be accepted in experimental work. In 1920, he and R. Rayner published an account of how they had induced fear of a white rat in Albert, an 11-month-old child, by the linking several times of the appearance of the rat with a sudden loud noise.[1] Little Peter was luckier. He became frightened of a rabbit because another child had shown fear of it. Mary Cover Jones (1924) introduced the rabbit to him at gradually lessening distances while he was having his elevenses so that he learned to associate the rabbit with something pleasant, and with, it could also be said, the relief of something unpleasant — hunger.[2]

Ivan Pavlovitch Pavlov (1849–1936) was Professor of Physiology at St Petersburg and a former student of Wundt. His famous contribution to psychology was the conditioned reflex. In the early 1920s he was working with dogs. Salivation was the normal uncon-

*Professor Ivan Pavlovitch Pavlov*

ditioned reflex response to the offer of food. The appearance of the food then coincided with the ringing of a bell. After repetition, it was possible to elicit salivation by the ringing of the bell alone. The dog had been conditioned to make this reflex response. Pavlov then went on to explore what would weaken, strengthen or extinguish the conditioned reflex. He noted that animals of different temperaments differed in the ease with which they could be conditioned. In 1924, the year when Petrograd changed its name, Leningrad was flooded and in Pavlov's laboratory the dogs were nearly drowned. He discovered that those which had reached a state of collapse through being unable to tolerate the extreme fearful stress had lost their conditioned responses. From this came his concepts of cortical excitation and cortical inhibition.[3] Sargant and Shorvon, in their ether abreaction treatment of traumatic war neurosis already quoted, came to the conclusion that the best results were obtained when they had induced in the patient a state of excitement by suggesting true or even artificial memories of stress to the point where excitement was followed by emotional collapse: the anxiety responses conditioned by the original stress had been extinguished.[4]

In 1958 Joseph Wolpe, a South African, published in his book *Psychotherapy by Reciprocal Inhibition* the results of the work he had been doing in the previous ten years. Reciprocal inhibition — a term he borrowed from Sir Charles Sherrington's work on spinal reflexes — means that if a response antagonistic to anxiety can be conditioned to occur in the presence of a stimulus which usually evokes anxiety, then the anxiety will be weakened or suppressed and the bond between it and the usual stimulus will also be weakened. Thus, if anxiety, an unpleasant symptom of neurosis, was a conditioned response, his treatment method aimed at weakening and then extinguishing the conditioned response by replacing it with another conditioned response of a pleasant and acceptable nature. The pleasurable conditioning response was deep muscular relaxation and the patient had to learn first how to achieve it. A neurosis is more than one anxiety response to one particular stimulus. The manifestations of anxiety in Man are multiple and so are anxiety-producing situations. Wolpe got his patient to make a hierarchy of stressors, that is, a list of all situations which produced symptoms in him ranked from the mildest to the most severe. Then he presented the mildest situation to the patient using the muscular relaxation to weaken the anxiety. The presentation could be actual in the case of phobias of objects such as spiders or cats or snakes, or in the imagination in the case of situations such as fear of crowds or lifts or heights. When the mildest had been dealt with, treatment proceeded to the next one up the scale. This is called systematic desensitisation.

The principle of weakening the undesirable response by strengthening the desirable has been applied in several ways. Group desensitisation could be used for patients with the same problem, e.g. agoraphobia.

Anxiety relief was the linking of the anxiety to the cessation of an unpleasant sensation, a mild electric current. Little Peter learned his anxiety response from imitating another infant. Modelling, the imitation of another coping with the feared situation, can reduce anxiety.

The pad and bell treatment of nocturnal enuresis devised by Mowrer and Mowrer in 1938, consists of weakening the urination response by linking it to waking. Inhibition of the undesirable response ensures an undisturbed sleep. Of course, a conditioned response of anger to the sound of the bell can be established in the inhabitants of the terrace house next door.

Aversion therapy has been used in the treatment of alcoholism, sexual deviations and pathological gambling. In alcoholism, an emetic such as emetine or apomorphine was administered and timed so that the onset of nausea and vomiting coincided with the offering of the patient's preferred tipple. The same technique was used when sexual deviants were shown slides of the objects which produced sexual arousal. The drugs produced circulatory collapse in some patients and were so unpleasant for others that the treatment was abandoned. The averting stimulus was changed to electric shock of high voltage and low amperage. Some patients were provided with a portable shock apparatus so that they could reinforce the aversion if faced with temptation away from the clinic.[5]

Negative practice is the intensive voluntary repetition of an undesirable action such as a tic or habit spasm. Intense and prolonged repetition without reinforcement weakens the drive behind the act. Alternatively, a state of excitation is followed by a state of reactive inhibition. G. Wakeham in 1928 is credited with the first report of this method. He was irritated by the mistakes he made in the playing of Bach's Toccata and Fugue in D minor on the piano and he played the mistakes deliberately and repeatedly. In two weeks he had eliminated them and could play the piece faultlessly.[6]

Avoidance of the anxiety-producing situation or stimulus reinforces its effect. Flooding or implosion therapy negates reinforcement by preventing avoidance. There is the same grading of stressors as in systematic desensitisation but, in the latter, anxiety is relieved by the substitution of a relieving manoeuvre, whereas in implosion therapy the situation is continued until the anxiety reduces. It has parallels in the excitation and inhibition of negative practice and abreaction.

B.F. Skinner was one of the learning theorists — others are C. Hull, O.H. Mowrer and H.J. Eysenck — who greatly influenced behaviour therapy. His 'operant' is a behavioural act which is desired. In operant conditioning, undesirable behaviour is ignored or disapproved; desirable behaviour is rewarded.[7] It has been applied in the treatment of autistic children and the mentally handicapped. Another example is the token economy of a ward for long-stay patients in a mental hospital. A patient whose personal care improved, who helped in the running of the ward, who joined in occupational activities and who increased his interaction with others was rewarded with tokens which would get for him desirable things such as cigarettes, sweets, entertainment, privileges. At first the desirable behaviour was immediately rewarded. The improved patient could proceed to the next stage where he would be paid on pay day and would have to budget for his tokens to last until next pay day. Subsequent stages signalled greater initiative and independence. Undesirable behaviour would attract fines.[8]

A well known example of the token economy was at the Institution for Criminal Psychopaths at Herstedvester in Denmark, of which the first Director was Dr Georg Sturup. In addition to individual therapy in which the individual's present interpersonal conflicts were related to his previous criminal behaviour, there was a system of rewards and gradings. Transgressions would mean a slither down the snake. Improvements earned progress up the ladder.[9]

Like other forms of treatment, behaviour therapy is not applicable to all psychiatric problems. Desensitisation and implosion are more suited to neuroses which are marked by relatively narrow ranges of anxiety manifestation and those in which symptoms of autonomic imbalance predominate. Operant conditioning is more suitable for behavioural problems in which there is some proportion of voluntary control.

# References

1. Gelder M.G. (1979). Man of Controversy. *British Medical Journal*; **279**:1416.
2. Beech H.R. (1969). *Changing Man's Behaviour*, Chapter 2. Harmondsworth: Penguin.
3. Pavlov I.P. (1927). *Conditioned Reflexes*. London: Oxford University Press.
4. Shorvon H.J., Sargant W. (1947). Excitatory abreaction. *Journal of Mental Science*; **93**:709.
5. Beech H.R. (1969). *Op.cit.* Chapter 10.
6. Wakeham G. (1938). Query on 'A Revision of the Fundamental Law of Habit Formation'. *Science*; **68**:135.
7. Skinner B.F. (1938). *The Behaviour of Organisms*. New York: Appleton-Century-Crofts.
8. Atthow J.M., Krasmer L. (1938). In *Abnormal Psychology*. (Maher B., ed.) pp.391–404. Harmondsworth: Penguin.
9. Sturup G.K. (1948). The management and treatment of psychopaths in a special institution in Denmark. *Proceedings of the Royal Society of Medicine*; **41**:765.

# III: Environmental and Social Treatment

## CHAPTER 9

# *The Evolution of the Mental Hospital*

Man interacts with his surroundings. If, as a patient, he is being adversely affected by his setting, change it or remove him to a better one. If he is having a bad effect on the setting, improve him or remove him from it to a place of safety. These considerations may prompt a pilgrimage to a healing shrine, changes in household or occupation or dwelling place, the prescription of a holiday or a long journey, confinement or admission to a hospital for treatment.

## The early hospitals

The link between religion and healing which was established in the pre-Christian temples was carried over into the Christian and Moslem civilisations of Europe and the Near East. A monastery would be not only a place of prayer and work and contemplation but could have a herb garden and an infirmary and an out-patient dispensary. In one of his letters, Alcuin (735–804), the tutor of Charlemagne who retired to become the Abbot of Tours, described the preparation of herbal medicines in the monastery.

The legend of the martyrdom of St Dymphna by her incestuously minded father dates back to the seventh or eight century and her shrine at Gheel in Belgium to the eleventh century. In the thirteenth century, there was a hospital there devoted chiefly to the care of mental patients.

The temple of Aesculapius on the island of the Tiber was succeeded by a monastery and hospital. It was there that Rahere (d. 1144) was ill and had the vision which led to his founding of St Bartholomew's Hospital at Smithfield. The medieval hospitals anticipated the modern district general hospital in accepting psychiatric cases as well as others.

Bethlem Hospital, founded in London in 1247 as the Priory of St Mary of Bethlehem, can claim to be Britain's mental hospital with the longest continuous history.

In the Moslem world, the Asclepion temples in Anatolia were succeeded by hospitals, and between the eighth and thirteenth centuries there were special facilities for the mentally ill in Baghdad, Damascus, Aleppo, Cairo and Fez. A mental hospital was built in Granada in 1365, and two stone lions now in front of the Ladies Tower in the Alhambra came from there. The treatments available in these places included special diets, baths, perfumes, drugs and concerts. At the Al-Mansur Hospital in Cairo there were storytellers to soothe the sleepless.[1]

## The madhouses

At the Dissolution of the Monasteries, Bethlem Hospital became the responsibility of the City of London and at the end of the sixteenth century was starting to receive patients from outside London. There was no other institutional provision for the mentally ill until private madhouses began to appear in the next century. Families who could afford to pay would board their sick relatives with a doctor or a clergyman or other willing person, some of whom opened establishments to take a number of patients. The conditions in which the patients would be kept varied with the psychiatric views, the facilities, the scruples and the business sense of their keepers. James Carkesse, a clerk at the Admiralty, wrote *Lucida Intervalla* in 1679 describing in doggerel his experience in Dr Thomas Allen's madhouse in Finsbury and later in Bethlem, of which Samuel Pepys, his superior, was a governor.[2] Daniel Defoe, in 1728, wrote on the abuses in madhouses but it was not until 1774 that a regulating Act was passed.

Of the three doctors in charge of King George III in his second attack of mental illness, two — Rev. Dr Francis Willis (1718–1807) of Lincoln and Anthony Addington (1713–1790) — were the proprietors of private asylums. The other two leading mad-doctors of the time, William Battie (1703–1776) of St Luke's Hospital and John Monro (1715–1791) of Bethlem, also ran private establishments. Charles Lamb spoke in praise of the private madhouse in Islington where his sister Mary was held several times, and William Cowper was an inmate of Dr Nathaniel Cotton's Collegium Insanorum at St Albans in 1763. After recovery, he stayed a further 12 months. In contrast, there were others where the patients were manacled to the wall and slept on straw.[3]

## The hospitals in the eighteenth century

This century, the Age of Enlightenment, saw the origin of many of the hospitals which have formed the foundation of the present services, although provision for the mentally ill was made more slowly than for the general sick.

At the beginning of the century, Bethlem Hospital was the only psychiatric hospital in Britain. In 1724, Bethel (House of God) Hospital was founded at Norwich under the will of Mrs Mary Chapman for the poor inhabitants afflicted with lunacy.

When Thomas Guy's Hospital was opened in 1728, four years after his death, he had specified separate provision for 20 lunatics, being those who had been discharged from St Thomas' or Bethlem or any other hospital without hope of cure. In 1733, Bethlem followed suit by building two wings for 100 incurable patients.

Public subscribers established St Luke's Hospital at the other side of Moorfields from Bethlem in 1751 and William Battie was its first physician. His *A Treatise on Madness* (1758) was based on his clinical experience rather than on speculation and he pointed out that there could be spontaneous recovery without treatment and that the vigorous purging and emesis then fashionable could be harmful rather than curative. This drew from John Monro across the way *Remarks on Dr Battie's Treatise on Madness* in which, among other things, he said that Dr Battie's attack on bloodletting was 'no less destructive than a sword'. These differences of opinion apparently did nothing to impair the collaboration of the two men in committee (Battie was a governor of Bethlem), in consultation and in the courts.[4]

Another who had become a governor of Bethlem in 1714 was Jonathan Swift, author of *Gulliver's Travels*. He was concerned about the possibility of becoming insane and mentioned it in his *Verses on the Death of Dr Swift* in 1731. When he died in 1745 he left money to found a mental hospital, and St Patrick's Hospital was opened in Dublin in 1757. In his own words:

He gave the little wealth he had
To build a home for fools and mad
And showed by one satiric touch
No nation wanted it so much.

In Newcastle-upon-Tyne, a Lunatic Hospital was opened in 1767, a private one, St Luke's House, having been opened in 1764.[5] The trustees of the Public Infirmary in Manchester, which was opened in 1752, were prevailed upon to build an addition for 'Poor Lunaticks which was opened in 1766 and enlarged in 1787 and again at the beginning of the nineteenth century. Its success as an adjunct to the Infirmary was quoted by Dr James Currie (1756–1805) when he was campaigning for a similar foundation in Liverpool — which was opened in 1790 and had a keeper and a matron from St Luke's Hospital in London. The latter had developed a fine reputation, not only for the quality of the care given by the head man keeper Thomas Dunston and the head woman keeper his wife, but also because Dr Battie had admitted medical students and doctors to attend lectures and observe the practice of the hospital. James Monro (1680–1752), predecessor and father of John Monro at Bethlem, had refused to do this.

The first mental hospital in Scotland was the Montrose Lunatic Hospital founded in 1781 by Mrs Susan Carnegie. It became the Royal Scottish Asylum in 1811 and has recently celebrated its bicentenary.[6]

One indication of the increasing interest in mental hospitals is the account in 1789 by John Howard (1726–90), the penal reformer, in which he compared Bethlem, St Luke's and St Patrick's with 'two Hospitals for Lunatics' at Constantinople, the Narrenturm at Vienna built by the Emperor Josef II in 1784, the Asylum at Frankfurt and the Madhouse at Amsterdam which was closed in 1792, although to Howard it had seemed to be the best he had seen. What he approved of in Amsterdam and Constantinople was that the rooms led on to open corridors and gardens, not passages as in Britain.

In an Appendix to his *Chapters in the History of the Insane in the British Isles*, to which all subsequent writers on the subject are indebted, Daniel Hack Tuke (1827–95) lists 15 hospitals making provision for mental patients in 1792, the year of the founding of the York Retreat. At that time public interest was being increased by the illnesses of George III, and eventually an Act of Parliament in 1808

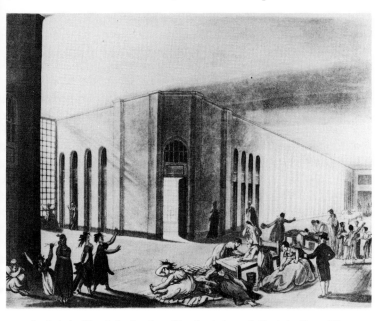

*St Luke's Hospital, London (Rowlandson and Pugin). From* The
Microcosm of London *1809*

(Wynn's Act) authorised counties and boroughs to join with private
subscribers to build mental hospitals for pauper and private patients.
The statutes of the General Hospital at Nottingham, founded in
1781, forbade the admission of mental patients, but the governors
started laying money aside for a separate foundation. They were
quick off the mark when the 1808 Act was passed and the new
asylum was opened in 1812, being equal first with Bedford's.

## Abuses and reforms in the eighteenth century

The mentally sick, unless protected by wealth or a strong caring
family or humane legislation, have always been at a disadvantage. In
an age which accepted poverty, pain and public executions as com-
monplace, it is not surprising to find that they were badly treated.
Although there is evidence of private kindness and public charity
towards them, it is the unkindness and neglect which has held the
attention of historians.

The conditions in which the patients in Bethlem were kept were well known, not only from the written accounts of the visitors such as Pope, Richardson and Walpole, but also because of the practice of admitting the public to view the patients as an entertainment. In 1749, William Hutton, a stocking weaver, walked from Nottingham to London and saw St Paul's and the King's house for nothing. He could not afford anything else except 'one penny to see Bedlam was all I could spare'. In the hospital he met 'a multitude of characters' and heard 'a variety of curious anecdotes'.

Hogarth painted the eighth scene of *The Rake's Progress* in 1733 showing the Rake in Bethlem's ward for incurables. In the background were two visitors, a lady and her maid. This and Goya's two paintings *La Casa de Locos* and *El Corral de Locos*, done at the prompting of his friend the poet and asylum reformer Melendez Valdes, are the only major works depicting the plight of the insane before the nineteenth century. Delacroix later pursued the same theme of the patient as an object of curiosity in his *Tasso in the Madhouse*. The abolition of public visiting at Bethlem in 1770, while merciful in one way, left the patients without any witnesses of their treatment or ill-treatment. The insane were also a public spectacle at the Bicêtre in Paris and as many as 2000 Parisians would flock there on a Sunday.[7]

York Lunatick Asylum was founded in 1777 'on a charitable foundation, with, it cannot be doubted, the best intentions on the part of its promoters, but, unfortunately, its management had been no better than the worst asylums of that day.' (D.H. Tuke). In 1791, the friends of Hannah Mills, a Quaker confined there, were refused admission to see her before she died and the suspicion of ill-treatment could not be allayed. The consequence of this was that in the next year William Tuke (1732–1822), a tea merchant, moved by this and by the experience of seeing patients at St Luke's lying on straw and in chains, persuaded the Society of Friends to establish 'an asylum openly conducted and on humane principles'. The Retreat was opened in 1796. The name was proposed by Daniel Tuke's grandmother to signify a place of refuge, a quiet place of withdrawal from the world.

Samuel Tuke (1784–1857), grandson of William and father of Daniel, wrote a *Description of the Retreat* in 1813 in which he told how his grandfather had personally managed it during the first years. Dr Thomas Fowler, whose arsenical solution was still in the pharmacopoeia in the twentieth century, was the first doctor and Samuel

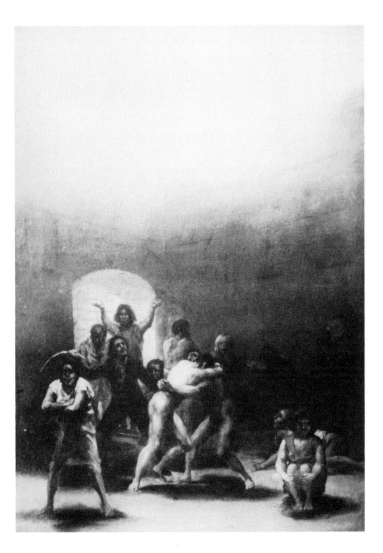

*Goya: El Corral de los Locos*

Tuke described how he tried and discarded as useless the bleeding, setons and evacuants which were currently recommended. Contrary to the practice of reducing patients by semi-starvation, he fed the excited ones well with plentiful supplies of porter 'always avoiding, in all cases, any degree of intoxication . . .' The principles of moral, by which is meant psychological, treatment were stated to be: strengthening and assisting the patient to control his disorder, using restraint only when absolutely necessary; and applying measures to improve the general comfort of the patients. An important factor in applying this last principle was to grade and separate the patients so that the more disturbed patients did not upset the quiet ones, a practice not always followed in modern establishments. Discipline and good behaviour were insisted on but chains or corporal punishment could neither be used nor could their use be threatened. Rather was self-restraint encouraged by an atmosphere in which loss of esteem of others was something to be concerned about.

When William Tuke gave up the management of the Retreat and became Secretary and Treasurer, his duties devolved on George Jepson and his wife Katherine who served there for 26 years. The hospital was always 'open to the inspection of intelligent enquirers' when others concealed their practices behind closed doors.

William Tuke's great contemporary in France was Phillipe Pinel (1745–1826). He had been in Paris since 1778, although he did not practise medicine for the first few years. In the 1780s, he started to take an interest in mental illness and in August 1793, seven months after he had witnessed the execution of Louis XVI, he was appointed the physician to the Bicêtre, the public mental hospital. Appalled by the conditions which he found there — one patient had been chained up for 40 years, another for 36 — he applied to the Commune for permission to unchain the patients. That body was very suspicious that enemies of the people were being concealed in the Bicêtre, and Couthon, the President, went on a personal inspection. The curses and abuse of the patients did nothing to appeal to his libertarian views but he grudgingly gave permission.[8] One of the grateful patients, an ex-soldier named Chevigné, attached himself to Pinel as a bodyguard and repaid him by saving him from a revolutionary mob who would have hanged him for harbouring priests and *emigrés*.[9]

In 1795, Pinel moved to the Salpêtrière and continued his reforms. His introduction of case histories and progress notes laid the founda-

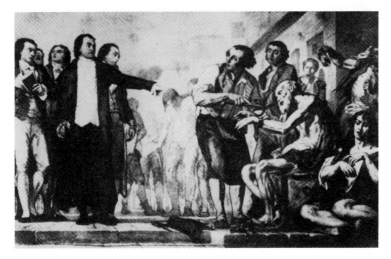

*Pinel liberating patients at the Bicêtre. Mural painting by C. Muller in the*
*Salle Bader, Académie de Médécine, Paris*

tion of the classifications and description of mental illness embodied in his *Traité-Medico-Philosophique sur L'aliénation mentale* in its second edition of 1809. He opposed bloodletting, the ducking of patients and the indiscriminate use of drugs. The staff were forbidden to strike patients, even if provoked, and were dismissed if they disobeyed. Convalescent patients were recruited to look after their less fortunate brethren. Pinel did believe in the influence of fear and other pressures: threats would be made but not carried out, ridicule of delusional ideas would be employed, a patient could be 'sent to Coventry' until his behaviour improved or have a cold douche to allay excitement.

Another contemporary reformer was Vincenzo Chiarugi (1759–1820) who was appointed Superintendent of the Hospital of Bonifazio, built by the Grand Duke, Pietri Leopoldo of Tuscany, in 1788. He laid down that patients should be treated humanely, restraint should be minimal, physicians should visit the wards daily, and there should be a programme of recreation and therapeutic work. Work for the hospital could only be prescribed by a physician. Hygiene and comfort were of great importance. His insistence on tact and understanding, on authority being wielded in a pleasant way, on the patient being respected as a person is the essence of the moral treatment.[10]

## Conditions in nineteenth-century hospitals

The publication of Samuel Tuke's book in 1813 moved the officers of the York Asylum to write sharply and combatively to the press. This had the opposite effect to that intended: local people started to investigate the Asylum and Friends like William and Samuel Tuke paid £20 to become governors, uncovering abuses which led to the dismissal of all the staff and the commission of Mr and Mrs Jepson ro reorganise the Asylum.

The discovery of James Norris in Bethlem by a visitor, Edward Wakefield (1774–1854) in 1814 led to another public outcry. Norris had been confined for 14 years and was enclosed in a device of bars going round the waist with projections to anchor his arms, bars over the shoulders and a ring round his neck. This was chained to the wall and his right leg was chained to the trough in which he lay.

A Parliamentary Select Committee 'Appointed to consider of provision being made for the better regulation of madhouses in England' was set up in 1815 as a consequence of these discoveries. Mr Godfrey Higgins, JP (1773–1833) described how he had discovered at York Asylum, behind a door which he was told was locked and of which the key had been lost, four cells in a dreadful condition of filth in which 13 women were confined in areas of eight square feet. A total of 365 patients had died but only 221 deaths had been reported.[11] William Tuke at the age of 83 was called on to give evidence about the running of the Retreat. He described the use of leather belts and the strait waistcoat rather than the straitjacket for restraint and the value of the warm bath for calming a patient. The Committee heard that at Bethlem there were two male and two female keepers for 52 male patients and 68 females, that Dr Thomas Monro (1759–1833), son of John Monro, attended once in three months and that the straw was changed once a week. There were 14 to 20 patients in chains. When the witness was asked what proportion of patients were naked or nearly so, he said that there were a good many but they were fewer now. Dr Monro said 'We do not administer medicines in the winter season; because the house is so excessively cold it is not thought proper'. In a private madhouse in Wiltshire, 13 of 14 patients were fettered and all but 3 were confined in cells which had no windows.

The Rev. J.T. Becher of the visiting committee of the Nottingham Asylum told the Select Committee that there were 16 patients of the

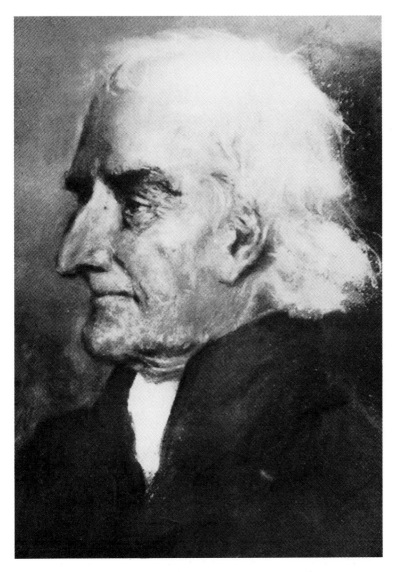

*William Tuke 1732–1822; portrait by H. S. Tuke*

first class, i.e. wholly paid for by relatives; 20 of the second class who were supported partly by relatives and partly by charity; and 40 paupers who were a charge on their parishes. There were three male and three female keepers, one of each for each class of patients. When he was asked if one keeper was equal to looking after 20 patients, he replied 'Twenty patients are seldom found without some in a state nearly advancing to recovery, and with a disposition in the case of any emergency to assist the keeper'.[12]

In spite of the findings of the Select Committee, no legislation ensued. Bills to make better provision for the regulation of madhouses were thrown out by the House of Lords in 1816 and 1819.

Further evidence of miserable conditions for pauper lunatics was given to Parliament in 1823 and 1827 but it was not until 1845, following a damning report by the Metropolitan Commissioners in Lunacy (they were established by an Act of 1828 to replace five useless Commissioners appointed by the College of Physicians), that Lord Ashley (1801–85), better known as the seventh Earl of Shaftesbury, the great philanthropist and social reformer, brought forward two Bills for England and Wales although, said he, 'I believe that not in any country in Europe nor in any part of America, is there any place in which pauper lunatics are in such a suffering and degraded state as those in Her Majesty's kingdom of Scotland'.[13] The importance of his second Bill was that it made the provision of county and borough asylums, permissive under the 1808 Act, mandatory.

In America, the influence of Pinel and William Tuke, rather than the practice of Benjamin Rush, had led to the foundation of such hospitals as the Bloomingdale Hospital, the Hartford Retreat, and the Friends Hospital at Frankfurt where humanitarian methods were used. At Frankfurt no chain was used, but, as at the York Retreat, leather was substituted for iron. Seclusion tended to replace mechanical restraint. Provision for mental patients was sparse and Dorothea Dix (1802–1887), a Massachusetts teacher who had visited the York Retreat, found a group of insane patients in a jail where she was conducting Sunday School. She investigated the situation in the jails and almshouses of the State and in 1843 presented a report to the State Legislature. After this she enlarged her activities and pressed on community leaders and legislators colourful reports of her findings. She is credited with influencing the foundation of more than 30 mental hospitals. In 1855 she visited the mental hospitals of Scotland and expressed great dissatisfaction with what she found there. An

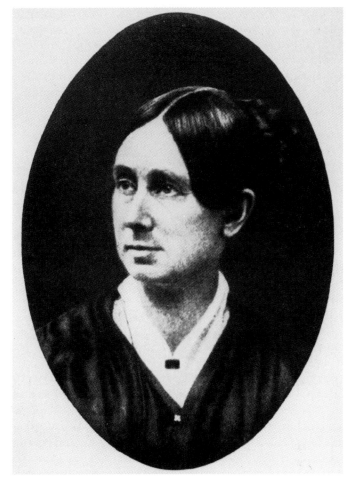

*Dorothea Lynde Dix*

official who planned to counter her opinions was shocked to find that she had caught the night mail from Edinburgh to London and had interviewed the Home Secretary while he was still on his way. The energetic intervention of 'the American Invader', as the Superintendent of Crichton Royal called her, resulted in the appointment of a Royal Commission which found conditions of restraint, seclusion in dark, unfurnished cells, cold, nudity and deprivation of light. Legislation followed in 1857 and the Home Secretary was moved to regret that the reform was due to 'a foreigner, and that foreigner a woman, and that woman a dissenter'. That the movement for reform endured was shown by the 1881 Report of the Commissioners in which they devoted 14 pages to recent changes: the abolition of walled airing-courts, the open-door system, liberty on parole, the removal of restrictions, industrial occupation, increased comfort, the boarding-out of lunatics, etc.[14]

## Restraint and non-restraint

The brighter side of hospital psychiatry in early decades of the nineteenth century comes out in the movement to abolish mechanical means of restraining excited, aggressive and overactive patients. The early reformers introduced a new atmosphere of kindness into asylums but did not forswear restraint. Pinel described coercing a patient first by the use and then merely by the possible use of a 'little velvet waistcoat'. Guillaume Ferrus (1784–1861), a surgeon in Napoleon's Grande Armée and later Physician-in-Chief to the Bicêtre, visited the Retreat in 1826 and found that a belt was employed, softly padded, to which the arms were attached.

Johann Gottfried Langerman (1768–1832) was the Director of the first mental hospital in Germany, St Georg at Bayreuth, from 1805 to 1810, and abolished restraint and the straitjacket; but non-restraint was not generally accepted in Germany until the 1860s when Connolly's book had been translated. The prime mover in Britain was Edward Parker Charlesworth (1783–1853), physician to the General Hospital at Lincoln and visiting physician at Lincoln Lunatic Asylum (later The Lawn). The Rules of this latter institution laid down that 'the patients be treated with all the tenderness and indulgence compatible with the steady and effectual government of them' and the staff were to behave 'with the utmost forbearance, tenderness and humanity to the unfortunate sufferers entrusted to their care'. These words are also to be found in the Rules of the Nottingham Lunatic Asylum and indicate a common source — Brislington House near Bristol, founded by the Quaker Dr Edward Long Fox (1760–1835). From about 1820, Charlesworth gradually reduced the use of 'padded iron collars, heavy leather muffs, iron wristlocks and leg locks', required that every use of restraint be recorded and, following the death of a patient in a straitwaistcoat in 1829, ruled that an attendant must remain in the room when a restraint was used during the night.

Pl. XIII

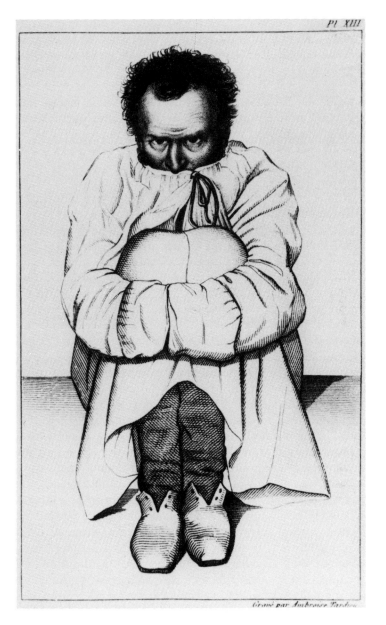

*Restraint by straightjacket. Plate 13 from Esquirol's* Des Maladies
Mentales *1838, and reproduced in Morison's* Physiognomy of Insanity
*1840*

In 1834, there was a period of several days when no restraint was used.[15] In 1835, Robert Gardiner Hill (1811–78) was appointed Resident House Surgeon and, after making statistical tables, comparing different modes of treatment and reflecting on the ability to dispense with restraint for days at a time, '. . . I announced my confident belief that under a proper system of surveillance, with a suitable building, instrumental restraint was in every case unnecessary and injurious. I mentioned this opinion to Dr Charlesworth and the Governors; I adopted it as a principle; I acted upon it; and I verified my theory by carrying it into effect.'

This quotation is from the lecture which Hill gave at the Lincoln Mechanics Institute on 11th May, 1838.

From 323 instances in 1835, restraint was reduced to 39 in 1836, 3 in 1837 and nil in 1838. Later Hill met such opposition from inside and outside Lincoln that he felt compelled to resign his post, but the reform which he and Dr Charlesworth had initiated was not lost.

Mr Sergeant Adams, Chairman of the visiting justices at Hanwell, took an interest in other asylums when he was on circuit. He was impressed by what he saw at Lincoln and commended it to Dr John Conolly (1794–1866), who had been appointed to the physicianship of Hanwell. Conolly visited Lincoln before he took up his appointment on 1st June, 1839. In his first report to the Visitors on 21st September of that year, he announced the abolition of all forms of mechanical restraint. His views on psychiatry and its practices were embodied in several publications, the most influential of which was *On the Construction and Government of Lunatic Asylums and Hospitals for the Insane*, published in 1847. In this he laid down that an asylum should be on a healthy site with a school and a chapel, that it should not have high gloomy walls or narrow inaccessible windows and that it should be planned to allow for the accumulation of incurable patients. In his opinion, the optimum number of patients was 360–400. If there were more, the medical superintendent needed assistance. He should be to the patients 'their physician, their director and their friend'. The matron should be under the direction of the superintendent. Exercise, games, access to gardens, musical evenings and dances as well as employment should all be part of the patient's life. Of his other important innovation, he wrote in 1856 in *The Treatment of the Insane Without Mechanical Restraints*: 'At Hanwell, clinical teaching was commenced in 1842. It appeared to me that then only could the proper study of insanity begin; the removal of restraints, and of all violent and irritating methods of control, then first permitting the student to contemplate disorders of the mind in their simplicity, and no longer modified by exasperating treatment. Patients could then be presented to their observation as subjects of study and reflection, and not as criminals; and regarded as persons to be cured of illness, or relieved from distress, and not as beings to be tortured by confinement of the limbs, or modified by punishments. Scenes of general confusion and agitation, opposed to the possibility of study, had become rare; the wards were tranquil, the patients were cheerful; and the visits of the pupils were looked forward to with interest. The actual state of the minds of the insane was in most cases easily displayed to the learner, without the least distress to the patient'. (Sir) William Gull was one of the students who attended Conolly's clinical lectures.[16]

Conolly's non-restraint regime was followed at Northampton and Haslar and Lincoln and Montrose but others, such as Corsellis at Wakefield, defended restraint, and W.A.F. Browne at Dumfries warned that absence of restraint did not guarantee absence of cruelty. Andrew Blake, Visiting Physician to the Nottingham Lunatic Asylum, regretted that Conolly had done away with the coercion chairs: a few, well padded and with straps, should have been retained for infirm and paralytic patients. It was at Nottingham that the First Annual Meeting of the Association of Asylum Superintendents took place in 1841. The Association, which became in 1865 the Medico-Psychological Association, in 1926 the Royal Medico-Psychological Association, and in 1971 the Royal College of Psychiatrists, passed at that meeting a resolution covering different shades of commitment: 'That without pledging themselves to the opinion that mechanical restraint may not be found occasionally useful in the management of the insane, the Members now present have the greatest satisfaction in according their approbation of, and in proposing their thanks to, those gentlemen who are now engaged in endeavouring to abolish its use in all cases'.[17]

Non-restraint was not received uncritically outside Britain. The French were sceptical, especially Ferrus who described how he had seen four powerful attendants holding down a furious epileptic in Conolly's own hospital. Isaac Ray (1807–81), the American whom his contemporaries regarded as the embodiment of his own dream figure, *The Good Superintendent*, forthrightly declared at a meeting of the Association of Medical Superintendents that non-restraint might work with Europeans who were accustomed to obey orders but no with Americans who believed in liberty and would assert themselve even when insane. The difference in views continued into this cen tury, when English psychiatrists argued that wet packs were a forn of restraint and American psychiatrists claimed that they used then as a calming therapeutic measure.

In 1879, Henry Maudsley (1835–1918), Conolly's son-in-law, wa attacking the too free use of sedatives which he called 'chemica restraint',[18] and in his 1881 Presidential Address to the Medico Psychological Association, Daniel Hack Tuke quoted the opinion o others that 'while the bromide has slain its thousands, chlora hydrate has slain its tens of thousands'.

In recent years too, there has been criticism of chemical restraint The value of the neuroleptics is to relieve the patient's distres sufficiently to make him responsive to the therapeutic and socialisin; influences of the hospital environment. Overdosage produces a quie but unresponsive patient.

## The retreat into custodialism

This is a phrase borrowed from an American writer which describe the changed pattern of psychiatric hospital care in the second half o the nineteenth century.[19] In the USA, population growth and the immigration of large numbers of foreign poor led to the demand fo: larger hospitals. Through the efforts of Dorothea Dix, patient; previously in gaols, almshouses and with their families were bein; admitted to hospital and many of these had chronic illnesses. Unti 1856, the Association of Medical Superintendents had, following the opinion of Thomas Kirkbride (1809–83), who was one of thei; founders, held out for a maximum of 250 beds in a state hospital Under pressure, they assented to a 600-bed policy but that did no; remain long when New York built the Willard State Hospital o. 1500 beds, and larger ones followed.

In England the 1845 Act was followed by the opening of 12 asylums in the next two years, and in 1854 there were still te; counties unprovided for. There was great opposition to the capita expenditure as well as to the maintenance costs. At Northampton where the private hospital, later St Andrew's, became no longer abl; to take the county's pauper patients on contract, critics of the lavisr expenditure on the new County Lunatic Asylum were mollified b;

he discovery that the running costs were reduced by taking in patients from other asylums which were full and the profits ensured hat 'the Northampton ratepayer will not again be called on for the money' for any alterations or extensions.[20]

The changeover from private philanthropy through private plus public concern to wholly public provision for the insane which had taken place since the beginning of the century, together with the increase in the population and the urbanisation accompanying the industrial revolution, increased the pressure on facilities. Existing asylums were extended and new ones were planned to house larger numbers. Economy of scale appealed to those who had to find the money. The warnings of earlier years were disregarded. John Reid (1776–1822), physician to the Finsbury Dispensary, wrote in 1816: 'Many of the depots for intellectual invalids may be regarded only as nurseries for and manufactories of madness . . .',[21] and in 1859 John Thomas Arlidge (1822–99), a pupil of Conolly, wrote 'In all cases admitting of recovery . . . a gigantic asylum is a gigantic evil'. He said that asylums had grown into lunatic colonies of 800, 900 or even more than 1000 inhabitants. The economic and administrative advantages were offset by the fact that the medical staff was not proportionately increased. No medical officer could look after up to 500 patients, give proper attention to the newly admitted and recent cases and also attend to the details of management which were necessary to ensure successful moral treatment. 'In a colossal refuge for the insane, a patient may be said to lose his individuality, and to become a member of a machine . . .' As W.A.F. Browne put it: 'In the vast asylums now extant . . . all transactions, moral as well as economic, must be done wholesale'.

In spite of Conolly's efforts, the number of patients at Hanwell, built to house 500 in 1831, increased from 800 to 1000 in a few years and in spite of his views on the appropriate size of an asylum, when Middlesex County Council built their second one at Colney Hatch in 1851 they provided 1200 beds. J.M. Granville in 1877 described it as 'a colossal mistake' and wrote of long, narrow, gloomy wards, oppressive corridors, a dingy atmosphere, and prison-like airing courts. He gave a similar account of Hanwell, adding that the gatekeeper was attired like a gaoler and that the male attendants displayed the same forbidding uniform.[22]

The growth is shown by the figures on the following page.[23]

|      | Average no. of patients per asylum | No. of county and borough asylums |
|------|------|------|
| 1827 | 116  | 9  |
| 1890 | 902  | 66 |
| 1910 | 1072 | 91 |
| 1930 | 1221 | 98 |

Pliny Earle (1809–92) of the Northampton Lunatic Asylum, Massachusetts, pointed out, in 1876 in his *Curability of Insanity*, how over a period of 30 to 40 years the percentage of reported recoveries in US asylums had dropped from 46% to 34%, and he suspected that the figures were being made to look better by basing them on patients discharged, not on patients admitted. He also advocated the separation of curable from incurable patients and quoted the favourable opinion of his German colleagues whom he had visited. Similar views were held by Edward James Seymour (1796–1866), physician to St George's Hospital and Metropolitan Commissioner in Lunacy, 1830–38. He proposed that milder cases should be treated at home and that patients should be discharged to home care before fully recovered. Samuel Gaskell (1807–1886), who was the Medical Superintendent of Lancaster County Lunatic Asylum and later Commissioner in Lunacy and who is commemorated in the Gaskell Medal and Prize of the Royal College of Psychiatrists, argued that mild recoverable mental illness would be treated better if patients could voluntarily opt for treatment in places less repugnant than lunatic asylums. This reform was included in the Mental Treatment Act of 1930, 70 years after he wrote.

The reports of the Commissioners in Lunacy give estimates of 11.2% curable cases in county and borough asylums in 1860 and 7.7% in 1870, and the cure rates for 1870, 1880, 1890 as 8.54%, 8.31% and 7.68% of total numbers resident. These contrast with the figure of 15.4% of pauper patients in county asylums estimated curable by superintendents in 1844.

One writer has suggested that the deterioration in standards was influenced by the increasing numbers of patients — up to 25% of male admissions in some asylums — with dementia paralytica. The relentless progress of dementia and death would have a dispiriting effect on the medical and nursing staff.[24]

## References

1. Baasher T. (1975). The Arab Countries. In *World History of Psychiatry* (Howells J.G., ed.), p.583. London: Baillière Tindall.
2. Hunter R.A., Macalpine I. (1963) *Three Hundred Years of Psychiatry 1535–1860*, p. 124. Oxford: Oxford University Press.
3. Allderidge P. (1979). Hospitals, madhouses and asylums: cycles in the care of the insane. *British Journal of Psychiatry*; **134**:321.
4. Doerner K., (1981). *Madness and the Bourgeoisie*, pp.39–47. Oxford: Blackwell Scientific Publications.
5. Le Gassicke J. (1965). The early history of psychiatry in Newcastle-upon-Tyne. *British Journal of Psychiatry*; **120**:419.
6. Presly A.S. (1981). A Sunnyside Chronicle 1781–1981. Montrose: Sunnyside Royal Hospital.
7. Jones C. (1980). The new treatment of the insane in Paris. *History Today*; October 1980.
8. Zilboorg G. (1941). *A History of Medical Psychology*, p. 319. New York: W.W. Norton.
9. Reeves J.W. (1958). *Body & Mind in Western Thought*, 'History has it that during this period Pinel successfully persuaded the authorities to unchain the mental patients in the Bicêtre. Drama has it that one of them subsequently saved his life from the Revolutionary mob.'
10. Mora G. (1975). *World History of Psychiatry*, Howells J.G. ed. pp. 62–5. London: Baillière Tindall.
11. Tuke D.H. (1882). *Chapters in the History of the Insane in the British Isles*, p. 151. London: Kegan Paul.
12. Jones K. (1955). *Lunacy, Law and Conscience*. London: Routledge, Kegan Paul.
13. Tuke D.H. (1882). *Op.cit.*, p.185.
14. Tuke D.H. (1882). *Op.cit.*, p.339.
15. Leigh D. (1961). *The Historical Development of British Psychiatry*, Vol. 1, *18th and 19th centuries* Oxford and London: Pergamon.
16. Leigh D. (1961). *Op.cit.*, p.224.
17. Walk A. (1970) Lincoln and Non-Restraint. *British Journal of Psychiatry*; **117**:481.
18. Maudsley H. (1879). *The Pathology of Mind*. London: Kegan Paul.
19. Tourney G. (1971). Psychiatric therapies 1800–1968. In *Changing Patterns in Psychiatric Care* (Rothman T., ed.) p.10. London: Vision Press.
20. Scull A.T. (1979). *Museums of Madness*, p.217. London: Allen Lane.
21. Hunter R.A., Macalpine I. (1963). *Op.cit.*, p.1025.
22. Scull A.T. (1979). *Op.cit.*, pp.193, 195, 198.
23. Jones K. (1960). *Mental Health and Social Policy*. London: Kegan Paul.
24. Hare E.H. (1959). The origin and spread of dementia paralytica. *Journal of Mental Science*; **105**:594.

CHAPTER 10

# The Development of a Mental Health Service

## The advance is resumed

While asylums were becoming larger, there were voices raised to plead for the separation of early curable cases and their treatment in small units. In 1851, Dr J.G. Davey, one of the superintendents of the megalopolis of Colney Hatch, had proposed a hospital of no more than 250 beds for the insane poor of London. The idea of 'small is beautiful' was revived in the 1880s when Dr Strahan of Northampton County Asylum proposed a hospital of 30 beds for curable cases only, attached to each asylum. Reception houses, for observation and short-term treatment, were advocated on the lines of one successful in Australia, and the psychiatric unit at the Charité Hospital in Berlin was also cited as a model. The latter and those in Munich and Göttingen inspired the foundation by voluntary effort of the Lady Chichester Hospital in Hove in 1905. Out-patients were seen there by Dr Helen Boyle and mild recoverable cases admitted. In the Presidential Address to the Medico-Psychological Association in 1889, Dr Hayes Newington repeated the theme, and when he became Chairman of the East Sussex Asylums Committee he was able to have a hospital villa built at Hellingly Asylum. Others followed.

The London County Council, urged by Mr Brudenell Carter, who was an ophthalmic surgeon at St George's Hospital and who was influenced by the views of Dr (later Sir) John Batty Tuke MP on the curative approach, adopted a report recommending the provision of a Reception House and then went on to build 2000-bed hospitals at Bexley and Horton. In 1895 the Council had appointed

Dr (later Sir) Frederick Walker Mott (1853–1926) to be the first Director of a mental hospital pathology laboratory at Claybury. He visited Kraepelin's clinic at Munich and returned with the idea of a university psychiatric clinic devoted to early treatment, research and postgraduate education. He used the preface of his research report, *Archives of Neurology*, in 1907, to put forward his scheme and linked it with the scheme for a Receiving House, which the London County Council had just abandoned after a fruitless seven years spent in trying to promote an enabling Bill. Henry Maudsley, whose pupil Mott had been at University College, London, then offered through Mott £30 000 to the London County Council to build such a hospital provided that it was associated with the University. His offer was accepted in 1908 but the site on Denmark Hill was not chosen until 1912 and the buildings were not completed until 1915.[1] Mott moved his laboratory there from Claybury in 1916 and during the First World War the Army and the Ministry of Pensions were in occupation. The Maudsley Hospital opened in 1923. Only non-certified patients could be admitted, the Council having obtained Parliamentary approval for this in 1915 so that 'many patients suffering from incipient mental disease would be induced to offer themselves for treatment who would otherwise not do so'.

The first Medical Superintendent was Edward Mapother (1881–1940). He had come into psychiatry in 1908 as a *locum tenens* at Long Grove Asylum which had opened in the previous year. Although the first Mapother Lecturer at the Institute of Psychiatry, Sir Aubrey Lewis, who was Mapother's successor there, says 'It may be safely assumed that from this date he had resolved to make psychiatry his life's work', the fact that he passed the Primary FRCS examination in 1909 and the Final in 1910 suggests that his original intention was to take advantage of the ample free time available to asylum medical officers to complete his studies. The lightness of the duties was an attraction for convalescents and aspirants to higher qualifications and others not primarily interested in psychiatry. Ernest Jones was familiar with that scene before he gave his allegiance to Freud and in his reminiscences he quotes a superintendent who said of his new assistant medical officer 'I don't expect him to be interested in insanity but he must be able to play cricket with the patients'.[2]

At Long Grove, Mapother came under the influence of a most enlightened superintendent, Dr (later Sir) Hubert Bond (1870–1945), and the keen young men who had joined his staff. Bond had a minimum of locked doors, shrubberies instead of walls and fences, no seclusion, and halfway houses for convalescent patients, measures which Mapother took with him to the Maudsley Hospital when he went there in 1919 to work for the Minstry of Pensions. When it was formally opened by the Ministry of Health in 1923, Mapother told the press that 'it is the first institution of its kind to be founded in Great Britain on the lines of the neurological and psychiatric clinics of the Continent and America, designed for the combined treatment and investigation of organic nerve diseases, neuroses and incipient psychoses'.[3]

Neuroses and incipient psychoses were suitable for out-patient treatment and a clinic had been opened at St Thomas' Hospital by Dr Rayner of Hanwell as early as 1889; another by Dr P. Smith at Charing Cross Hospital followed and other early examples were those of Dr Edwin Goodall at Cardiff and Dr Thomas Beaton at Portsmouth.[4] In 1910, Dr Oswald of Gartnavel established an out-patient clinic at the Western Infirmary, Glasgow. After its closure during the 1914–18 War, it was re-opened by Dr (later Professor Sir) David Henderson with the help of a social worker and a psychologist.[5] Sir David was one of the most distinguished pupils of Adolf Meyer (1866–1950), the great leader of American psychiatry who taught a psychobiological psychiatry and advocated a comprehensive mental health service. The Mental Treatment Act of 1930 empowered the local authorities to set up out-patient psychiatric clinics, and the medical staffs of their mental hospitals started to come out into the community and reach the patients with non-psychotic illness. The Feversham Report indicated that there were 166 out-patient clinics in England and Wales in 1936.

The other big advance in the 1930 Act was the provision of voluntary status for patients so that the stigma and legal disability of certification were avoided. The knowledge that one could discharge oneself having given up to three days notice was another advancement. Further encouragement to voluntary admissions was given when hospitals built new separate accommodation for their reception and the newer physical treatments were becoming available. Personal accounts of the psychiatry of this era have been written by both authors of the seminal text *An Introduction to Physical Methods of Treatment in Psychiatry*, William Sargant and Eliot Slater.[6,7]

Advances in the mental hospitals were checked between 1939 and

1945 by shortages of medical and nursing staff, drafting of caring relatives into war work and the taking over of mental hospital beds for the Emergency Medical Service. The slowing up of treatment and rehabilitation and the overcrowding led to an accumulation of unimproved patients, normal maintenance had been neglected and planned improvements had been shelved.

The first notable advance was the open-door policy. Open doors were not new. At Fife and Kinross Asylum in the 1870s, Dr John Batty Tuke (not a member of the York family) had open doors, and Woodilee Asylum in 1881 was nearly all open. One thing which had militated against a policy of freedom was that until 1924 every escape of a patient had to be notified to the Board of Control. Several hospitals had one or two open wards in the 1930s, but during the Second World War opinion turned again and the doors swung shut. The three men who revived open doors were Dr George Bell of Dingleton Hospital, Melrose, who had an open hospital by 1949,[8] Dr Duncan Macmillan of Mapperley Hospital, Nottingham, who accomplished the opening of his wards between 1949 and 1952 — Pinel took six years to unfetter all his patients — and Dr T.P. Rees at Warlingham Park Hospital, Croydon, who finished opening a year later.[9] By 1956 the Ministry of Health reported that seven hospitals in England were without locked wards.

Re-education of the nursing staff to a therapeutic rather than a custodial role and a programme of active treatment of new patients and rehabilitation of others were pre-requisites for success. The community had to be prepared to accept the new measures by informative contacts between staff and public and by visits of interested bodies to the hospitals. The results were an improved atmosphere in the hospital, marked lessening of tension, and a considerable reduction in disturbed behaviour with a consequent disappearance of the need for seclusion. Padded rooms were dismantled: the Stanley Royd Hospital at Wakefield was very pleased in 1979 to be given materials salvaged from another hospital to enable the reconstruction of a padded room in its Museum.

The conversion of certified patients to voluntary status often resulted in a change of attitude in the long-stay patient and his family and was the beginning of a successful rehabilitative process leading to discharge. Certification was avoided for disturbed and uncooperative admissions by the use of a short-term (3 and 14 days) observation order which gave time for treatment to have an ameliorating effect so that, if necessary, the patient could continue in hospital as a voluntary patient. In 1955, there were 1370 admissions to Mapperley Hospital: only one (from prison) was certified and 79 were on short-term observation and discharged within that time.[10] Other hospitals could similarly claim over 90% admissions of voluntary status.

When the National Health Service started in 1948, the mental hospitals passed from the management of the local authorities to Regional Hospital Boards. Visiting Committees, who had to be concerned with how much money they asked from the ratepayers who elected them, were succeeded by Hospital Management Committees who, encouraged by medical superintendents and senior staff, could make a case for increased expenditure without that constraint. The enhanced financing provided better staffing, structural and decorative improvements and a general raising of hospital standards in catering, furnishing and recreation. Social security benefits now ensured that patients had pocket money and could acquire personal clothing and belongings. The reduction of overcrowding gave increased comfort and also gave space for new therapeutic facilities.[11]

Similar changes were slower in occurring in the USA, although in the 1950s the mental hospitals of Britain had many visitors from there. In 1962 it was possible to say that while there were some open hospitals, camisoles, cuffs and wet packs were still used in some American hospitals.[12]

## Work therapy

Galen (AD 130–201) said 'Employment is nature's best physician and is essential to human happiness'. For him, employment was anything by which a skilled or unskilled worker earned his livelihood.

Occupation was an important part of moral management. At The Retreat 'the advantage of regular labour in some cases' was recognised, and Bucknill and Tuke, in their *Manual of Psychological Medicine*, echoed Chiarugi in saying that '. . . no lunatic patient should be permitted to engage in work except under medical sanction. Asylum stewards and bailiffs ought to be kept under strict control in this matter'.[13]

Sir William Ellis, at Wakefield and then at Hanwell, relied on occupation for his patients. They had the incentive and satisfaction of

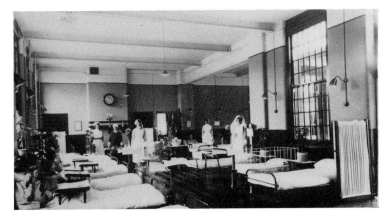

*Mapperley Hospital, Nottingham: a ward in the 1930s*

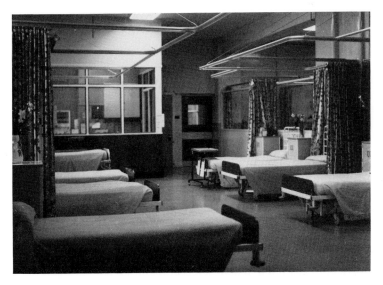

*The same ward in the 1980s*

earning something and, recognising that poverty and unemployment were potent factors in causing relapse, Ellis had some patients taught a trade. He could say at Hanwell that 454 out of 610 patients were employed. At Wakefield he had had to overcome opposition to the idea: one suggestion was that each patient allowed outside to work should be chained to a keeper; another was that a corner of the garden should be reserved for the patients and they should dig it over and over again.

In 1838, Samuel Tuke was preparing to edit the translation of Jacobi's *On the Construction of Asylums* and he visited Scotland. He found the wards of the asylums at Perth, Dundee and Aberdeen empty during the day as the majority of the patients were employed. At about the same time W.A.F. Browne was saying at Montrose 'The whole secret of the new system and of that moral treatment by which the number of cures has been doubled may be summed up in two words, kindness and occupation'.[14] In the first Medical Superintendent's Report for 1880, Dr Evan Powell told the Visiting Committee of the new Nottingham Borough Asylum 'Special prominence has been given in the treatment of patients to employment'.

Special prominence was given to employment in the 'More Active Treatment' promoted by Dr Hermann Simon (1867–1947) of Gutersloh in Germany in the 1920s. His persistence with the most regressed and withdrawn patients produced results and his methods were widely copied in Western Europe. A lot of what Simon did was not new to those who had not forgotten Ellis and his successors. The typical mental hospital was a large community (a word used by Ellis) and its patients helped to run it. There was work for the men on the farm and in the gardens and for the women in the sewing room and the laundry. The cook, the plumber, the tailor, the joiner, the shoemaker and other tradesmen could have patient helpers and the responsibility of supervising them was recognised with a small addition to their wages.

Nevertheless, the enthusiasm engendered by Simon induced The Board of Control to circulate a report on Occupational Therapy for Mental Patients in 1933 (HMSO) and Dr Ivison Russell of Clifton Hospital, York, wrote a book about it.[15] The first School of Occupational Therapy was opened at Dorset House in Bristol in 1930 by Dr Elizabeth Casson OBE. It moved to Bromsgrove during the Second World War and then settled at the Churchill Hospital in Oxford. The Association of Occupational Therapists was formed in 1936 and incorporated in 1943. It set its first public examinations in 1938. The term 'occupational therapy' conjures up the image of craft work, but contact with the profession brings a diversity of activities into the picture: music, games, play reading, art classes, quizzes, relaxation sessions, domestic management, etc. All these are means to the ends of treatment: distraction from morbid preoccupation; deflection or diversion of unacceptable drives; prevention of progressive impairment; maintenance of normal personal, social and work habits; encouragement of those personality traits which will protect from future breakdown.

When the rehabilitation of patients with chronic mental illness was being undertaken in the revitalised hospitals after the Second World War, it was realised, following Ellis, that employment after discharge would help prevent relapse. It was also realised that the nineteenth century methods of preparing patients to return to an agricultural and lightly industrialised society would not suffice. Industrial therapy was introduced and it developed in a variety of forms.[16] A simple example was at Cheadle Royal (the successor to the Manchester Lunatic Hospital) where the patients produced Christmas novelties. The choice of this product was made because it was cheap, no capital outlay for machinery was involved and the manual labour of the patients was unlikely to be replaced by automation.[17] At Banstead Hospital in the industrial unit the men did piece-work for a car factory and the women assembled cardboard boxes.[18] At Netherne Hospital the potentiality of patients for industrial therapy was assessed at a weekly conference which was attended by the Disablement Resettlement Officer of the Ministry of Labour. A patient could be allocated to employment in the hospital or at the local Industrial Rehabilitation Unit. Such patients lived in a halfway house where they took much responsibility for their own management.[19]

The limitations of hospital workshops were discussed in a King's Fund Report of 1968, when those in 100 hospitals were reviewed. Criticisms were that the work lacked variety, the patients learned no new skills, their earnings were low and the work bore no relation to the needs of local industry. This last point was not entirely valid: local firms provided work on contract for the industrial units. Of the working hours reviewed, 61% was devoted to unskilled bench and assembly work — folding, labelling, gluing, stapling — whereas only 0.2% comprised skilled woodwork. It was noted that more depressed than schizophrenic patients were discharged from the units but twice as many schizophrenics were discharged via the units as direct from hospital.[20]

In 1955 the Medical Research Council sent two psychiatrists and a psychologist to study rehabilitation methods on the Continent. They found that in Holland the influence of Dr Simon had not waned. In the psychiatric rehabilitation unit of Dr P. Sivadon at Ville Evrard near Paris, there were 250 beds but the unit had twice as many doctors and three times as many nurses and social workers as the rest of the 850-bed mental hospital which housed it. Dr Sivadon claimed that the higher cost was offset by the higher discharge rate and shorter patient stay.[21] Similar cost-effectiveness was found by a social scientist and an accountant when they compared the resources and results of three hospitals in England in 1958.[22] In Dr Sivadon's unit work was graded according to the patient's capabilities. The most regressed worked at a primitive level on rubble crushing and crude clay modelling. The most skilled work to which patients could progress was in the printing shop.

An approximation to working conditions outside the hospital was first devised by the Industrial Therapy Organisation (Bristol). This started in the late 1950s when Dr Donal Early of Glenside Hospital realised that psychiatry knew little of industry and industry knew nothing of psychiatry. Lectures and talks to interested bodies such as Rotary, Chamber of Commerce etc. had produced no result. It needed a personal approach to an industrialist by the psychiatrist with a commercially viable proposition. The introduction of industrial supervisors ensured that correct production methods were used and that quality control was maintained. The nursing staff learned something of industrial methods and the supervisors learned something of patient management. The suspicion that patients were being exploited was overcome by inviting a Trades Council delegation, who reported that the work was therapeutic and that the venture should be supported. The next step, which required much hard work and negotiation, was to set up a factory outside the hospital. Employers seeking workers were more likely to look for them in a factory than in a hospital. The formation of a limited liability company, the recruitment of a knowledgeable Board of Directors and the obtaining of finance and of suitable premises were all settled within a relatively short time, and the combination of voluntary and hospital enterprise had achieved what the statutory powers of local authority

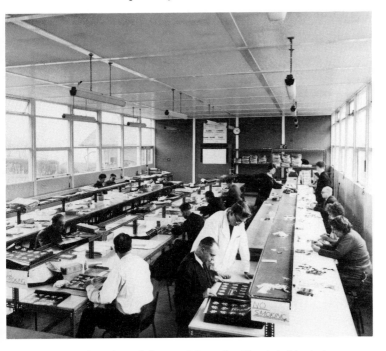

*Day unit for industrial therapy; Mapperley Hospital, Nottingham*

and Ministry of Labour had not.

'Of 673 referrals, ITO (Bristol) placed 174 patients in open employment in its first seven years and 129 in sheltered employment. Nearly one-quarter of those placed in open employment had been in hospital longer than ten years.'[23]

ITO (Thames) Ltd started after helping St Bernard's Hospital Re-employment Training Unit to expand. With a grant from the King Edward Hospital Fund, an interest-free loan from the Ministry of Labour, Ministry training allowances and hostel accommodation from Middlesex County Council, it was possible to open a factory in Hanwell in 1964 for 15 trainees whose total time in hospital added up to 320 years. Trainees came from St Bernard's, Springfield and Shenley Hospitals, after assessment by the Disablement Resettlement Officer (DRO). After 6 to 12 months work, the services of the DRO would again be used to place the ex-patient with a suitable employer.[24]

'This type of set-up cannot be run by committees; it is therefore, all important that some one person, preferably an industrialist, is found who will be willing to keep a constant and watchful eye on the day-to-day running of the company, and who has the confidence of the Board, and a free hand on industrial matters.'[25]

## Treatment in the community

The movement of treatment outside the mental hospital, which was interrupted by the Second World War, was resumed in the late 1940s and the ideal of a comprehensive mental health service was pursued by Dr Thomas Beaton in Portsmouth, Dr Francis Pilkington in Plymouth, Dr Duncan Macmillan in Nottingham, Dr J. Carse in Chichester and Dr W.A.L. Bowen in York. The list is not comprehensive. All these services had common characteristics: they were mental-hospital based; they accepted that the treatment of mental illness is a long process, that there must be continuity of care and that the sojourn as an in-patient is but one phase; pre-admission screening was as important as after-care; co-operation with community agencies was necessary; good public relations had to be established and maintained.

From Graylingwell Hospital, Chichester, Dr Carse set up 'The Worthing Experiment' in 1957. The establishment of a day hospital, out-patient clinic and domiciliary consultation service reduced the admissions from Worthing by 59%.[26]

The services in Portsmouth, Nottingham and York featured a close liaison with the Mental Health Departments of their local authorities. The duly authorised officers — those empowered under Section 20 of the Lunacy Act 1890 to arrange emergency short-term admissions — acted as social workers in the assessment of patients before admission to hospital or referral to the out-patient clinic and in home-visiting after discharge from hospital. They had no formal training but their practical experience was augmented by informal instruction in meetings at the hospitals and in telephone consultations and home visits with consultant psychiatrists.[27] When the 1890 Act was replaced by the Mental Health Act of 1959, they became mental welfare officers and their invaluable contribution to the services continued. The fruitful partnership between the local authority and the mental hospital was dealt a severe blow when the Seebohm Report of 1968 was followed by the Social Services Act of

1970. The creation of the generic social worker in the community meant the disappearance of the mental welfare officer with the expertise and the interest to help the mentally ill. The social worker, who was expected to deal with problems of the homeless, child care, the blind, the deaf, the elderly, the physically disabled, could scarcely be expected to welcome the problems of maintaining the mentally disabled in the community. The competing claims of all these categories of clients forced directors of Social Services to draw up orders of priorities. In one such list the mentally ill were not last: the mentally handicapped came after them.

The municipal social psychiatric service set up by Dr A. Querido in Amsterdam in the early 1950s was an interesting example of community treatment. The prominent feature was a crisis intervention team of doctor, nurse and social worker who would deal with the patient on the spot and then arrange to continue treatment as intensively as necessary in the patient's own home.[28]

The comprehensive mental health services as described here functioned because they dealt with well-defined and compact communities. For Salford, Dr H.L. Freeman refined the concept further by having a psychiatric team in the mental hospital designated as being in charge of all patients from that portion of the catchment area and relating to the social workers, local authority services and general hospitals of that area.[29] This resembled the Dutchess County Project in New York State in which a community was identified with a 550-bed unit set up in 1960 within a 5000-bed state hospital and which provided continuity with pre-admission screening and after-care clinics.[30]

Lancashire, with large mental hospitals serving distant populations, had some of its problems solved by the Manchester Regional Hospital Board which set up psychiatric units in general hospitals. In Blackburn, for example, the in-patient beds were backed up by out-patient clinics, an occupation centre, an industrial workshop, a therapeutic social club, a branch of Alcoholics Anonymous and a day centre.[31] Similar services functioned in Bolton[32] and Oldham.[33] By 1955, nearly half of all psychiatric admissions were to the small psychiatric units attached to general hospitals, yet these had only 20% of the total psychiatric beds. Patients treated in their own community could be more readily returned to it.

Day hospitals were for treatment. Day centres provided occupation. The day hospital at Worthing had a programme which included

ECT, modified insulin treatment and abreactions. Hospitals of later date could also provide individual psychotherapy, occupational therapy, group psychotherapy and group activities.

A therapeutic social club for in-patients at Runwell Hospital was started by Dr Joshua Bierer, who was a follower of Adler, in 1938 and this was followed by one for out-patients and discharged patients. Psychotherapy on a group basis and the socialising influences of refreshments and games and cultural pursuits were features. After the War, the work continued in the Social Psychotherapy Centre in Hampstead and the Marlborough Day Hospital.[34] When the idea was taken up elsewhere, its continued success depended on the commitment of the club leader, whether psychiatrist, social worker, occupational therapist or ex-patient.

In addition to the mental welfare officers there were social workers employed by the mental hospitals. In Nottingham, for instance, four social workers paid by the hospital worked from the premises of the Mental Health Department and formed a unified team with the mental welfare officers under the direction of the mental health officer.[35] Before the Social Services Department came into being in 1971, they withdrew to the hospital premises and were taken over as a functioning department by the Social Services, thus preserving their expertise for the benefit of the patients. Psychiatric social workers had been introduced to Britain by the Commonwealth Fund of America. The first were trained in the USA and worked in child guidance clinics here. In 1930 the first English course in social work began at the London School of Economics. The prevailing psychiatric doctrine outside the mental hospitals was psychodynamic, and psychiatric social workers grew up without a knowledge of the phenomena and management of acute and chronic mental illness, a disability inherited by the generic social worker. Physical treatments were equated with assaults on the patient and psychotherapy was thought to be the only genuine treatment. Away from London and university centres, psychiatric social workers were rare birds, and mental hospitals had to find and train their own social workers. A few had certificates in social work, some had moved out of mental nursing, others were just well motivated. What they lacked in theory they tended to make up in practical common sense.[36]

It was not long before the mental hospital psychiatrist was followed into the community by the psychiatric nurse. From 1954 at

Warlingham Park Hospital, Dr Rees had some nurses seconded to full-time extramural duties in the Borough of Croydon, and at Plymouth nurses' home visits increased from 740 in 1957 to 2878 in 1964. A survey showed that by 1967 nearly 50 hospitals were employing community psychiatric nurses. In some places this arose because of a lack of social workers, but it was soon recognised that the nurse could exert an influence not available to the social worker or mental welfare officer. The chronic psychotic patient resettled in the community responded better to the nursing approach, and the nurse could mediate between the patient and the warden or landlady of the hostel or explain the vagaries of the patient's behaviour to family or neighbours. Advice on continued medication came more readily from the nurse and was more readily accepted.[37] When the depot neuroleptics came into use, the work of the community nurses increased. In good psychiatric establishments there were no demarcation disputes. A conference of the psychiatric team could decide whether the nurse, the social worker or the mental welfare officer known to the patient would be the most suitable to undertake after-care.

Specific psychiatric treatment and the re-educative and resocialising influences of the hospital milieu resulted in numbers of long-stay patients becoming well enough to live outside hospital. Those without a welcoming family were settled in lodgings or hostels. Although the National Health Service Act had laid the obligation on local authorities to provide living accommodation for the homeless and helpless, little was provided and hospitals tackled the problem in various ways. Lodgings were found and patients boarded out with landlords and landladies. Unless the boarding houses and hostels were supervised, the patients could be neglected and drift into apathy and deterioration. It was necessary to provide social work support or nursing visitation and daytime occupation for the patients, and again, in default of local authority provision, the hospitals set up day centres either in the community or on hospital premises. These day centres also relieved the burden on families, and separate psychogeriatric day centres were especially useful in helping families to continue to care for their aged failing relatives. Voluntary agencies such as the Guideposts Trust and the local branches of the National Association for Mental Health (now MIND) provided homes in which small groups of patients could live together, helped by the visits of a voluntary worker and a community nurse. Early failures taught the hospitals that the patients for group homes had to be carefully selected for compatability and then trained to live together and share the household duties.

The methods of the comprehensive mental health service were particularly suited to dealing with the growing problem of the elderly mentally ill. Notification of a problem to the Mental Health Department resulted in a joint visit of local authority mental welfare officer or social worker and psychiatrist. The home situation could be assessed and the problem defined. It might be dealt with by medication at home or day-patient attendance or short-term admission either for rehabilitation or to give the relatives a break.[38] Beds in some psychogeriatric wards were set aside and could be booked ahead to give holiday relief. If action was taken in good time, rejection was avoided. Once relatives were set in an attitude of rejection, none of these measures availed and it was not possible to keep the patient in the community.[39]

## Mental nursing

The link between religion and the treatment of the mentally ill which began in the temples of the ancient world and continued in the Christian era, shows up in the early history of mental nursing. In 1539 a Portuguese ex-soldier, Joao Cuidad (1495–1550), who had experience of being confined as a lunatic, took a house in Granada and gave shelter to the mentally ill and other outcasts of society. His followers formed the Order of the Brothers of Charity and he was canonised as St John of God in 1690. The Order spread throughout Europe and its members were looking after patients in France, Poland and Bohemia in the seventeenth and eighteenth centuries. Its Maison Libre at Charenton in Paris was closed by the Commune in 1795.

St Vincent de Paul (1580–1660) was a Gascon who was ordained priest in 1600. After being captured by corsairs and sold into slavery, he escaped to France. In Paris he turned the leper hospital of St Lazare over to the care of mental patients and founded lay organisations for charity and nursing and helped Ste Louise Marillac to found the Order of Sisters of Charity, who nursed female patients in Poland and Central Europe; their Grey Nunnery was caring for the insane in Montreal in the eighteenth century.

The Recollet Monastery in Quebec had six cells for insane women in 1717 and six for men in 1723. The transition from monas-

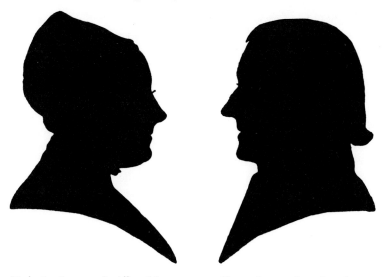

*Katherine Jepson, née Allen, Matron
and Female Superintendent at
The Retreat 1796–1823*

*George Jepson, Superintendent at
The Retreat
1797–1823*

tery to mental hospital also took place in Switzerland in the
nineteenth century after the defeat of the Sonderbund. St Pirmins-
berg became the psychiatric hospital for the canton of St Gallen.
Münsterlingen was converted from a monastery in 1848 and others
followed at Rheinau (Zurich) in 1867 and St Urban (Lucerne) in
1873. The monastery at Königsfelden, near Brugg, also became a
mental hospital.

John Haslam (1764–1844) was Apothecary to Bethlem from 1795
until he lost his post after the Report of the 1815 Select Committee
was published. He was one of the first to give some thought to
mental nurses and in his *Considerations on the Moral Management of
Insane Persons*, which he published in 1817, he drew attention to the
poor status and working conditions of the keepers and the dangers of
their work. He thought that they should receive instruction from the
doctors with whom they worked and that they should have a pen-
sion scheme, and a register of those suitable for the work should be
kept.[40]

Jean-Baptiste Pussin was already Governor — the equivalent of
chief male nurse — at the Bicêtre before Pinel was appointed. His
wife was Governess and they co-operated in Pinel's reforms. Other

husband-and-wife teams undertook or supervised nursing duties. Katherine Allen went from Brislington House to the Retreat and married George Jepson. Mrs Jepson's tea parties had a valuable socialising influence on the patients. Dr Samuel Hitch, Resident Physician at the Gloucester Asylum, had his wife appointed as Matron in 1838 — she had already looked after a disturbed child patient in her own home — and in 1841 the wife of the Charge Attendant was employed as a nurse in the refractory ward. Another superintendent's wife who took an active part in the care of patients was Mrs Ellis. When her husband, Dr (later Sir) William Ellis (1780–1839), was at Wakefield she organised the female patients into making useful garments and articles which were on sale to visitors. When her husband was appointed to Hanwell in 1831 she continued to act as matron and occupational therapist, and a report of a Fancy Fair at Hanwell Lunatic Asylum in the *Illustrated London News* in 1843 indicates that her influence lingered after they had left. William Ellis also called for better pay so that more respectable persons might be induced to become keepers and nurses after suitable instruction.

Samuel Gaskell at Lancaster was the first to employ a night attendant, thereby reducing the incidence of nocturnal incontinence.

The first formal instruction for nursing staff was a set of lectures given at the Surrey Asylum (Springfield) in 1843–4 by Sir Alexander Morison (1779–1866), the visiting physician. William Alexander Francis Browne (1805–85), father of Sir James Crichton-Browne, was appointed Medical Superintendent of the Royal Montrose Lunatic Asylum in 1834. 'What Asylums were, are, and ought to be' is the substance of five lectures delivered to the Managers there in 1837. This resulted in his being offered the superintendency of Crichton Institution in 1839 by its foundress, Mrs Elizabeth Crichton. In 1854–5, he gave a course of 30 lectures to the male and female attendants. Pleas for systematic training were unheeded by the Medico-Psychological Association until Dr Campbell Clark of the District Asylum, Bothwell, described the courses he had instituted in 1882. A committee was formed to consider training and instruction for attendants and the preparation of a manual. The first edition of *The Handbook for the Instruction of Attendants on the Insane* was produced in 1885. It was known, from the colour of its binding, as 'The Red Handbook' to generations of mental nurses until the demands of a wider syllabus rendered it old-fashioned. Classes were held in an increasing number of hospitals — 100 by 1889 — and in the next year the Association adopted a scheme of training, certification and registration. It was not long before between 500 and 600 nurses were qualifying for certificates each year. This was the first professional qualification in nursing. The General Nursing Council's qualifying examinations did not come into operation until 1925 and it was not until after the Second World War that the Royal Medico-Psychological Association agreed to the General Nursing Council's takeover of the examinations and registration of mental nurses.[41]

The first training school in the USA was organised at the McLean Asylum in 1882 by Edward Cowles and pupils were given a certificate on completion of the course. Training with a minimum course of instruction was standardised by the American Medico-Psychological Association in 1906.

Rules and regulations for nursing staff were strict. They had to live in the hospital if single and on the estate if married. A ward sister or a male staff nurse would have a bed-sitting room on or next to the ward. Nurses homes were a late addition to the hospital buildings. Off-duty periods could be as little as one day a fortnight. Misconduct could result in instant dismissal. Even as late as 1944, Rule No. 67 of the City Mental Hospital, Nottingham, stated that no nurse was allowed to marry without the sanction of the Visiting Committee.

The developments in the mental nurse's role are the outstanding feature of the history of treatment in the 1970s. Several influences have come together to produce far-reaching changes. The higher educational standards required of candidates for training have ensured that there are nurses who are capable of more demanding and more skilled work with patients. The pressure for psychiatric treatment means that psychiatrists have called on nurses for help with treatments which require individual attention. The taking over of parts of the nurse's job by social workers, occupational therapists and domestic supervisors has left clinical nurses dissatisfied. The expansion of services into the community now requires the application of nursing skills to maintain patients outside hospital and to apply treatments in the patient's home setting. Nurses are now trained in group therapy and behaviour therapy, and supply specialised services which previously were limited. Patients with phobias, with obsessive and compulsive neuroses, with sexual and marital problems — those conditions which can be crippling and which have gone untreated because they are time consuming — can now be given the concentrated attention which they need.[42]

# References

1. Walk A. (1976). Medico-Psychologists, Maudsley and the Maudsley. *British Journal of Psychiatry*; **128**:19.
2. Jones E. (1948). The early history of psychoanalysis. *Journal of Mental Science*; **100**:198.
3. Lewis A. (1969). Edward Mapother and the making of the Maudsley Hospital. *British Journal of Psychiatry*; **115**:1349.
4. Boyle A., Helen A. (1939). Watchman, What of the Night? (Presidential Address). *Journal of Mental Science*; **85**:859.
5. Harper J. (1959). Outpatient adult psychiatric clinics. *British Medical Journal*; **1**:357.
6. Sargant W. (1967). *The Unquiet Mind* London: Heinemann.
7. Slater E. (1975). Psychiatry in the Thirties. *Contemporary Review*; **226**:70. See also *Bulletin of the Royal College of Psychiatrists*, September and October 1981.
8. Bell G.M. (1955). A Mental Hospital with Open Doors. *International Journal of Social Psychiatry*; **1**:42.
9. Rees T.P. (1957). Back to moral treatment and community care. *Journal of Mental Science*; **103**:303.
10. Macmillan D. (1956). An integrated Mental Health Service; Nottingham's experience. *Lancet*; **ii**:1094.
11. *The Walls Came Tumbling Down — Mapperley Hospital 1880–1980*. Printed and published at Mapperley Hospital, Nottingham.
12. Clarke D.H. (1963). Administrative psychiatry 1942–1962. *British Journal of Psychiatry*; **109**:178.
13. Tuke D.H., Bucknill J.C. (1858). *Manual of Psychological Medicine*. London: Churchill.
14. Browne W.A.F. (1837). *What Asylums were, are and ought to be*. Edinburgh: Black.
15. Russell J. Ivison (1938). *The Occupational Treatment of Mental Illness*. London: Baillière Tindall & Cox.
16. Morgan R. (1974). Industrial therapy. *British Journal of Hospital Medicine*; February 1974:231.
17. Wadsworth W.V. (1958). A hospital workshop. *Lancet*; **ii**:896.
18. Baker A.A. (1956). A factory in a hospital. *Lancet*; **i**:278.
19. Bennett D.H., Folkards S., Nicholson A.K. (1961). A Resettlement Unit in a Mental Hospital *The Lancet*; **ii**:539.
20. Wansborough N., Miles A. (1969). *Industrial Therapy in Psychiatric Hospitals*. London: The King's Fund.
21. Carstairs, G.M., Clarke D.H., O'Connor N. (1955). Occupation treatment of chronic psychotics. *Lancet*; **ii**:1025.
22. Jones K. and Sidebotham R. (1962). *Mental Hospitals at Work*. London: Routledge, Kegan Paul.
23. Early D.F. (1968). The role of industry in rehabilitation. In *The Treatment of Mental Disorders in the Community*. (Freeman H.L., Daniel G.R., eds.) pp.25-33. London: Baillière Tindall, Cassell.
24. Green L. (1980). The factory with a difference *BMA News Review* Vol. 6, No. 10, October.

25. Turley J. (1965). *Notes for the Guidance of Those Interested in Setting up an Industrial Therapy Organisation*. ITO (Bristol) Ltd.

26. Carse J., Panton N.E., Watt A. (1958). A District Mental Health Service. *The Lancet;* **i**:39.

27. Pargiter R.A., Hodgson T.D. (1959). The M.W.O. and the psychiatrist. *The Lancet;* **ii**:727.

28. Querido A. (1955). The Amsterdam psychiatric first-aid scheme *Proceedings of the Royal Society of Medicine*; **48**:741.

29. Freeman H.L. (1968). The Local Authority and the Hospital Service. In *The Treatment of Mental Disorders in the Community*. (Freeman H.L., Daniel G.R., eds.), pp.34–8. London: Baillière Tindall, Cassell.

30. Gruenberg E.M. (ed). (1966). *Evaluating the Effectiveness of Community Mental Health Services*. New York: Milbank Memorial Fund.

31. Silverman M. (1968). Community medicine in relation to a comprehensive general hospital-centred psychiatric service. In *The Treatment of Mental Disorders in the Community* (Freeman H.L., Daniel G.R., eds), pp.58–67. London: Baillière Tindall, Cassell.

32. Leyberg J.T. (1959). A District Psychiatric Service; The Bolton Pattern. *Lancet*; **ii**:282.

33. Pool A. (1959). *The Organisation of Community Care for Oldham and District*. Paper read to Northern and Midland Division of RMPA.

34. Bierer J. (1948). Modern social and group therapy. In *Modern Trends in Psychological Medicine* (Harris N.C., ed.) pp.289–309. London: Butterworth.

35. Macmillan D. (1956). An integrated Mental Health Service: Nottingham's experience. *Lancet*; **ii**:1094.

36. Little J.C., Burkitt E.A. (1976). *Psychiatry and the Social Worker*. Welwyn Garden City: Smith Kline French Publications.

37. Baker A.A. (1968). Mental nursing in the community. In *The Treatment of Mental Disorders in the Community*. (Freeman H.L., Daniel G.R., eds.), pp. 6–14. London: Baillière Tindall, Cassell.

38. Silverman M. (1968). *Op.cit.*, p. 65.

39. Macmillan D. (1960). Preventive geriatrics: opportunities of a Community Mental Health Service. *The Lancet;* **ii**:439.

40. Leigh D. (1961) *The Historical Development of British Psychiatry* Vol 1. 18th and 19th Centuries, p. 124. Oxford & London: Pergamon Press.

41. Walk A. (1961). The history of mental nursing. *Journal of Mental Science*; **107**:1.

42. Bird J., Marks I.M., Lindley P. (1979). Nurse therapists in psychiatry. Developments, controversies and implications. *British Journal of Psychiatry*; **135**:321.

# CHAPTER 11

# *Conclusions*

The history of psychiatric treatment shows a continuous refinement with experience and the advance of scientific knowledge. The somatic treatments have almost entirely narrowed down from physical to pharmacological methods because a widening range of drugs has made possible a much more flexible and progressive regimen. Psychotherapy has moved on from the early rigid tenets of psychoanalysis to a varied pattern of approaches and techniques. New ideas in environmental and social treatment derive not only from the humane approach of the early reformers but from the experience and the freedom gained in somatic and psychological treatments.

Can we learn anything from this history or must we say with Aldous Huxley 'That men do not learn very much from the lessons of history is the most important lesson that history has to teach'?

One outstanding conclusion is that the history of psychiatric treatment shows up the complexity and variability of human nature. The subject is full of agreements and contradictions. Through it there runs a thread of charity. Be it called religion, humanism, enlightenment, enthusiasm, it finds expression in the commandment 'Thou shalt love thy neighbour as thyself', although it was expressed more often in action than in words. The pioneers and reformers showed it in their drive and persistence in the face of difficulty and disapproval. Their inner conviction sustained them often against the spirit of the time. Fray Juan Jofre founded Spain's first Christian mental hospital, El Hospital de Inocentes, in Valencia in 1409 as a protest against the stoning of a madman. Gardiner Hill at Lincoln singlemindedly pushed forward his assertion that restraint was unnecessary, even though a place of high reputation such as the Retreat still used it. There were glaring contradictions. Sir Thomas More (1478–1535), saintly in his personal and family life, 'the King's good servant but God's first', had a madman flogged into good behaviour. The Turkish Sultan who had his son strangled built a comfortable hospital for the mentally ill. Pinel unfettered the patients but adopted a severe attitude to those who would not conform to his methods of rehabilitation. Benjamin Rush helped found the first antislavery society in America, but his treatment methods were harsh. Even today there are doctors who, faced with a patient whose nervous system is torturing him with unpleasant sensations resulting from exposure to intolerable stress, will write out a prescription for a tranquilliser and an antidepressant and then advise the patient to 'throw all those tablets away' and go out and enjoy himself.

Another feature to be discerned in this history is the influence of chance, luck, inspiration, serendipity: call it what you will. Sir Charles Locock thought that he was treating hysteria with bromide and found an anticonvulsant for epilepsy. The convulsion treatment of melancholia resulted from a misconception of the biological status of epilepsy and schizophrenia. The first antidepressant was a failed neuroleptic. Cade was testing a hypothesis and found a treatment. Chlorpromazine was vindicated when the experimental dosage was increased, chlordiazepoxide when the dose was lowered. 'Chance favours only the prepared mind.' (Louis Pasteur). Advances are made by a refusal to accept the status quo. Medicine did not advance until knowledge later than that of the ancient authorities was required of candidates for medical degrees: the Rev. Francis Willis (1718–1807), who treated George III, was admitted to his medical degrees in 1759 after displaying only his familiarity with the works of Galen.

Each treatment in its day has had its staunch advocates and some have been more successful than others. In some cases success has led to excess. There have been sufficient examples of overenthusiastic purging, bleeding and drugging. Good results of ECT and leucotomy in well-selected cases were followed by poor results in patients less carefully selected. Unrewarding treatment has been persisted with because of the theoretical convictions — or stubbornness — of the therapist. Critics of psychotherapy can point to long courses of treatment without improvement. Exile from hospital into community care may be applied as policy rather than as the correct treatment for the individual. On the other hand, every worker in the mental health field can produce examples of surprises, of successful rehabilitation in most unfavourable cases, of victories achieved against the odds. This brings us back to the great variability of human nature and the possibility of the most unlikely adjustments. The lesson to be learned is that each patient is unique. What is desirable is a correct appraisal of the psychological, nervous and social factors in the illness and the correct choice of treatment. In some patients, drug treatment produces sufficient relief to enable them to solve their psychological and social problems; in others the psychological and social problems do not exist and their nervous symptoms are the response to previous stress. There are unhappy, distressed, maladjusted people who do not need drugs. Psychotherapy is indicated to help them adapt to life. In others, the correction of social problems and maladjustment is as important as either of the other two aspects. The wide span of the problems and the techniques required to solve them suggests that more than a single therapist is needed to cover them all. The modern concept of the mental health team, first seen in the child guidance clinics of the 1920s, has come into being to meet this need. Doctor, nurse, social worker, psychologist, occupational therapist, voluntary worker can each contribute special skills, but to the skills must be allied respect for the patient, respect for one's colleagues, and due optimism and humility in facing the task.

# Biographical and Historical Notes

Adler, Alfred (1870–1937)

> Born a Jew in Vienna. Became a Christian in adult life. Suffered from rickets in childhood. This influenced his choice of profession and his ideas on the effects of physical disability on the development of the personality. Qualified in medicine in 1895 and studied ophthalmology and industrial disease before going into practice.

> Although he resisted attempts to give Individual Psychology a specific religious bias, he was to lecture in Britain under the patronage of the Catholic Archbishop of Liverpool and the Anglican Archbishop of York. He died suddenly when visiting Aberdeen in 1937.

The Anatomy of Melancholy by Democritus Junior who was Robert Burton (1577–1640)

> Born in Leicester and educated at Nuneaton and Brasenose College, Oxford. From 1599 spent the rest of his life at Christ Church. Held livings in Oxford and Leicester.

> His book appeared in 1621 and deals with the causes, symptoms and cure of melancholy. It draws on Greek and Latin classics, the Bible and the Fathers of the Church and exhibits a wide range of curious learning. Sir William Osler called it 'the greatest medical treatise written by a layman'. Sterne borrowed some of the material for Tristram Shandy.

Avicenna (978–1036)

> Born in Bokhara, settled in Isfahan. Ethnic origin disputed by Persians, Turks and Arabs. His tomb is still a place of pilgrimage. He was appointed Court Physician at the age of 18. His

*Canon of Medicine* was in use as a textbook in Europe and the East as late as the seventeenth century.

Bethlem or Bedlam

Established 1247 in Bishopsgate by Simon Fitzmary as the Priory of St Mary of Bethlehem. Housed the insane by the end of the next century, passed to the City of London at the Reformation. Rebuilt at Moorfields in 1676 to the design of Robert Hooke, (1635–1703) MA, MD, FRS, horologist, physicist, inventor, microscopist. Transferred to Lambeth in 1815 where its building now houses the Imperial War Museum. Since 1931 the Hospital has been at Beckenham, Kent and it is now linked with the Maudsley Hospital.

Le Bicêtre Grange aux Gueux

Founded by Louis IX (1226–70) as a Carthusian monastery. In 1290 it passed to the Bishop of Winchester, of which Bicêtre is the corruption. Rebuilt after destruction in 1632. After being hospital and prison, became in 1610 a hospital for indigent and mentally ill men as part of the General Hospital of Paris.

Bleuler, Eugen (1857–1939)

Born near Zurich. Qualified in medicine 1883. Professor of Psychiatry at Zurich, 1898–1927. After early interest, became more and more critical of psychoanalytical theory. In 1911 he introduced the term schizophrenia for the group of disorders which Kraepelin had designated dementia praecox. Retired from Burgholzli at age 80.

Boerhaave, Hermann (1668–1738)

Professor of Medicine at Leyden. Introduced bedside teaching. Six of his pupils became professors at Edinburgh. Another, Gerhard van Swieten (1700–72), became Professor at Vienna, Court Physician to the Empress Maria Theresia, and Prefect of the Hofbibliothek.

Bond, Sir Charles Hubert (1870–1945)

Graduated at Edinburgh 1892. Psychiatric appointments at Edinburgh (Morningside), Wakefield, Banstead and Bexley. First medical superintendent at Long Grove 1907. Became a Commissioner of the Board of Control (1912) and eventually Senior Commissioner. Sued for wrongful detention by a paranoid patient in 1924. Bond and another doctor, believing him dangerous, had locked him in a room at the Board's offices. The case was set aside in the Court of Appeal and the House of

Lords. The patient accepted an out of court settlement in lieu of retrial. CBE, 1920. KBE, 1929.

Braid, James (1795–1860)

A native of Fife and a Member of the Royal College of Surgeons of Edinburgh. Became interested in mesmerism in 1841. Called it neurohypnotism and offered to read a paper on it to the British Association in 1842, but it was refused. Was opposed by Elliotson's followers in *The Zoist*. His hypnotic suggestion was introduced into France in 1859.

Cerletti, Ugo (1877–1963)

Became Professor of Psychiatry in Rome 1935. With Lucio Bini (1908–64), reported first results of ECT to Academy of Medicine, 15th March, 1938. In 1950 propounded theory of 'acroagonine', a substance produced in the brain by the action of ECT.

Charcot, Jean Martin (1825–93)

MD Paris 1853. Appointed physician to the Salpêtrière in 1862. Professor of Pathological Anatomy 1872. Professor of Neurology 1883. He was a great clinical observer, a dramatic lecturer and a talented artist.

Culpeper, Nicholas (1616–54)

Born in London. Practised in Spitalfields as an astrologer and physician. Fought in the Civil War on the Parliamentary side and was wounded. Pirated a translation of the *Pharmacopoeia* of the Royal College of Physicians. His *English Physician Enlarged*, a popular medical book, went into five editions before the end of the century.

Dix, Dorothea Lynde (1802–87)

Born in Maine of a drunken father and an indifferent mother. Brought up by grandparents in Boston. Trained as a teacher. Financial independence in 1837 enabled her to do reformist work. Visited the Retreat in 1836 and the mental hospitals of Scotland in 1855. In 1858, the Editor of the *Journal of Mental Science* reprinted, as a tribute, her 'Memorial praying a Grant of Land for the Relief and Support of the Indigent Curable and Incurable Insane in the United States' which she had presented to Congress in 1848.

Elliotson, John (1791–1868)

Became Professor of Medicine at London University in 1831. Founder and first President of the Phrenological Society. Was one of the first to use the stethoscope. Met Baron de Potet and became interested in mesmerism in 1837, and published in 1843 'Numerous cases of surgical operations without pain in the mesmeric state; with remarks upon the opposition of many members of the Royal Medical and Chirurgical Society and others'. Founded *The Zoist*, a journal to promote mesmerism in 1843, and a mesmeric hospital in Fitzroy Square in 1849. Thackeray dedicated *Pendennis* to him.

Ellis, Sir William Charles (1780–1839)

MRCS 1800. Practised in Hull. After making known his interest in mental illness by publishing a letter to a Member of Parliament, he was appointed the first superintendent at the Wakefield Lunatic Asylum. There he set patients to work, advocated moral management and allowed recovering patients to walk outside the hospital. He obtained the establishment of a charitable fund to help discharged patients. When he became the first superintendent of Hanwell in 1831, he carried over his enlightened ideas and the Queen Adelaide Fund there was set up at his inspiration. His beneficent regime made Conolly's improvements easy to introduce. He was knighted in 1835, the first psychiatrist to receive the accolade for his professional achievements.

Esdaile, James (1808–59)

Graduated MD Edinburgh 1830. Joined the East India Company and was in charge of a hospital near Calcutta. Impressed by Elliotson's claims he tried mesmerism and published the account of 100 operations done under its influence. Two medical committees of enquiry in 1846 and 1847 reported favourably on his practice. He continued this form of anaesthesia after the introduction of ether and chloroform.

Ferrier, Sir David (1843–1928)

Graduated in classics and philosophy at Aberdeen 1863 and in medicine at Edinburgh 1868. From 1871 at King's College, London, he was successively Demonstrator in Physiology, Assistant Physician, Consultant Physician and Professor of Neuropathology. FRS 1876.

Freud, Sigmund (1856–1939)

Born in Freiburg, Moravia. MD Vienna 1881. He carried out research in aphasia, in spastic diplegia and neuropathology. He studied cocaine and naively recommended its euphoriant properties for treatment of depression and morphine addiction. His colleague Carl Koller (1857–1944) discovered its local anaesthetic properties in Freud's absence. His Jewish blood and his sexual theories ensured that he was denied academic advancement and that he would be harassed by the Nazis. His friends conveyed him to London in 1938. Four of his sisters died in concentration camps.

Gerard, John (1549–1612)

A native of Nantwich. Admitted to the freedom of the Barber-Surgeons Company in 1569 and held office therein. He was superintendent of Lord Burghley's garden on the present site of St Martin-in-the-Fields and had his own garden in Holborn. His *Herball* of 1597 gives evidence of his knowledge of the history, preparation and uses of plants and practical knowledge of their cultivation.

*Gold-headed Cane, The*

A book by William Macmichael (1784–1839), physician to the Middlesex Hospital. The cane had a gold top containing aromatics to protect against infection. It was the symbol of the physician and was owned in turn by Doctors John Radcliffe, Richard Mead, Anthony Askew, William Pitcairn and Matthew Baillie. The cane's supposed biography is the vehicle for an interesting account of these five doctors. It was presented to the Royal College of Physicians by Matthew Baillie's widow.

Hall, Marshall (1790–1857)

A native of Nottingham and a graduate of Edinburgh. He demonstrated reflex action in the nervous system, campaigned successfully to abolish flogging in the army and introduced a method of artificial respiration. Was fiercely opposed to mesmerism.

Hippocrates (460–355 BC)

Born on the island of Cos and practised there and in Thessaly and at Athens. Died at Larissa. The collection of his aphorisms is obviously based on keen clinical observation. His high ethical standards find expression in the Hippocratic Oath.

Horsley, Sir Victor (1857–1916)

Qualified from University College Hospital, London, 1880. Superintendent of the Brown Institution, London, 1884–90 and did research on the thyroid gland, protection against rabies and the localisation of function in the brain. Assistant Surgeon, University College Hospital 1885 and Surgeon to National Hospital, Queen Square.

In 1887 successfully removed tumour from spinal cord. Devised an operation for the relief of trigeminal neuralgia. Professor of Pathology, University College Hospital 1887–96, Professor of Clinical Surgery 1896–1906. Knighted 1902. Died of heat stroke on active service in Mesopotamia.

Jackson, John Hughlings (1835–1911)

Born in Yorkshire. Medical education at York Medical School and St Bartholomew's Hospital and qualified in 1856. MRCP 1860. MD St Andrews 1860. Assistant physician and physician London Hospital 1863–94. Assistant physician to the National Hospital for the Paralysed and Epileptic, Queen Square 1862 and was on the active staff until 1906. FRCP 1868. Goulstonian lecturer 1869. Croonian lecturer 1880. Lumleian lecturer 1890. FRS 1878. He was a meticulous observer and an original thinker. The three fields in neurology for which he is famous are aphasia, epilepsy and the evolution and dissolution of the nervous system. Some of his observations on epilepsy were made on his wife who was a sufferer. His concept of levels of function in the nervous system influenced the thinking of psychiatrists, notably Adolf Meyer, W.H.R. Rivers and Henri Ey.

Janet, Pierre Marie Felix (1859–1947)

Born in Paris. Graduated in psychology and taught it before taking up medicine. Worked at La Salpêtrière towards the close of the Charcot era. Professor of Psychology at the Sorbonne 1898 and at the Collège de France 1902.

Jones, (Alfred) Ernest (1879–1958)

Born in Glamorgan. Qualified at University College Hospital, London, 1900. Thrice gold medallist. MD 1903; MRCP 1904; FRCP 1942. Director of Psychiatric Clinic and Associate Professor, Toronto 1908–12. Organised first psychoanalytic congress at Salzburg 1908. Private practice London 1913. Founder President British Psycho-Analytical Society 1919–44. Editor *International Journal of Psychoanalysis* 1920–39. Edited the first 50 volumes of the *International Psycho-Analytical Library*. Used his influence with the Home Secretary to obtain residence permit for Freud to settle in England and also helped other Jewish psychoanalysts to emigrate. Published three-volume

*Sigmund Freud*; *Life and Work* 1953–7.

Jung, Carl Gustav (1857–1961)

Son of a pastor. Worked at Burgholzli. 1906 Diagnostic Association Studies described his word–association tests as indicators of repressed material. His *Psychology of Dementia Praecox* was based on meticulous examinations of patients. He had an encylopaedic knowledge of mythology, philosophy and comparative religion and used it in developing his theories.

Kalinowsky, Lothar B.

Born 1899 of a Prussian father and Jewish mother and therefore unacceptable when the Nazis came to power. Took refuge first in Rome where he was present when the first ECT was given. Had to move to the USA where he introduced ECT into Pilgrim State Hospital, NJ. Became Clinical Professor of Psychiatry, New York Medical College.

Kraepelin, Emil (1856–1926)

Born at Neu-Strelitz, educated at Leipzig and Wurzburg, graduated in 1878. As a student he had written an essay on mental diseases for a competition. After working in physiological psychology with Erb and Wundt, he was successively Professor of Psychiatry at Dorpat (1886), Heidelberg (1890) and Munich (1904). The first edition of his textbook was published in 1883, the ninth in 1927. In the sixth edition in 1899 he drew together his own observations and those of his predecessors, Kahlbaum and Hecker, and classified the psychoses into two main groups: the manic-depressive and dementia praecox.

McDougall, William (1871–1938)

Born in Lancashire. Educated at Weimar, Manchester and Cambridge. Qualified from St Thomas' Hospital and worked with (Sir) Charles Sherrington in neurophysiology. After further study in Cambridge, Gottingen and London, he was elected Wilde Reader in Mental Philosophy at Oxford in 1903. His *Introduction to Social Psychology* in 1908 was widely acclaimed. During the First World War he served as a major RAMC. Appointed Professor of Psychology at Harvard 1920 and in his hormic or purposive psychology opposed Watson's behaviourism. His *Outline of Psychology* (1923) and *Outline of Abnormal Psychology* (1926) were very readable textbooks. Became Professor of Psychology at Duke University, N. Carolina 1927. FRS 1912.

Macewen, Sir William (1848–1924)

Diagnosed brain abscess 1876, successfully removed brain tumour 1878. Regius Professor of Surgery, Glasgow from 1892. A pioneer of bone surgery and thoracic surgery also.

*Malleus Maleficarum* 1488

Although demoniacal possession and the effect of witchcraft were put forward as the nature and cause of mental illness at various times from the beginning of history, it was the publication of this book, *The Witches Hammer*, which unleashed a widespread persecution of the mentally ill, the eccentric and the unfortunate throughout Europe. The authors were Heinrich Kramer and Jacob Sprenger, two Dominican theologians of Cologne. Not all accused of being witches and sorcerers were mentally ill but nearly all the mentally ill were considered to be so, or bewitched. The book went through 19 editions in three centuries. It provided guidance for the Inquisition and its influence was still active in the Salem Witch Hunt in the seventeenth century.

Mapother, Edward (1881–1940)

Born in Dublin, son of Edward Dillon Mapother, a surgeon. Qualified from University College Hospital, London, 1905. MD 1908; FRCS 1910. Served as a surgeon in Mesopotamia and France from 1914. Then worked at Maghull neurosis centre and 2nd Western General Hospital neurological division. Moved to Ministry of Pensions Hospital at Maudsley Hospital 1919. Member of the Child Guidance Council. Bradshaw Lecturer at Royal College of Physicians 1936.

Maudsley, Henry (1835–1918)

Born near Settle in Yorkshire. Educated at Giggleswick and privately at Oundle. Qualified from University College Hospital, London, 1855. Went to Wakefield for asylum experience preparatory to joining East India Company and stayed in psychiatry thereafter. After a spell at Brentwood, was appointed Medical Superintendent of Cheadle Royal at the age of 23. Physician to West London Hospital 1864. Editor of the *Asylum Journal* 1862–77. His *Physiology and Pathology of the Mind* (1867) was one of the major psychiatric works of the nineteenth century. President of Medico-Psychological Association 1871. Married Ann, younger daughter of John Conolly, and took over his Lawn House in 1866. Professor of

Medical Jurisprudence, University College, London, 1876. Gave £30 000 for the establishment of a mental hospital to be associated with the University of London. Also left legacy to the Medico-Psychological Association and is commemorated in the annual Maudsley Lecture.

Meduna, Laszlo (1896–1964)

Elaborated the technique of convulsion therapy at the Institution of Mental Care, Budapest, and published paper in 1935. Later moved to the USA where he promoted the carbon dioxide inhalation treatment of the neuroses in 1950.

Mesmer, Franz Anton (1734–1815)

Born near Lake Constance. MD Vienna 1766. Followed Richard Mead in believing that the gravitational attraction of the Sun and Moon, the recent discovery of Newton, had a periodic effect on the incidence of disease. Later was influenced by Maximilian Hell, Professor of Astronomy in Vienna, and treated patients by applying magnets. Results of stroking and making passes convinced him of the reality of animal magnetism. His wife was well connected and they had a prominent social position in Vienna and entertained Mozart at their home. Opposition forced his migration from Vienna to Paris. In France, founded the Society of Harmony with lodges in various towns. Suspicion of their political influence contributed to his expulsion from Paris.

Meyer, Adolf (1866–1950)

Born at Niederweningen near Zurich, the son of a pastor. He was a pupil of Auguste Forel (1848–1931) at Burgholzli. Studied in London, Vienna, Berlin, Paris and emigrated to the USA in 1892. Pathologist to New York Psychiatric Institute 1895–1902. Professor of Psychiatry at Johns Hopkins Medical School 1910–41.

In 1913, opened Henry Phipps Psychiatric Clinic where several distinguished British psychiatrists have studied. Gave the 14th Maudsley Lecture to the RMPA in 1933 on British Influences in Psychiatry, acknowledging his debt to Hughlings Jackson and Gowers and others.

Mitchell Silas Weir (1829–1914)

Born in Philadelphia. A pioneer neurologist who described nerve injuries in the American Civil War. His treatment of neurosis featured rest, isolation, abundant food, electrotherapy, exercises and massage as set out in his books *Rest in the Treatment of Disease* (1875) and *Fat and Blood* (1877). He also published poetry and novels and was critical of the political control of medicine and of the paucity of research in psychiatry.

Moniz, Egas (1874–1955)

Antonio Caetano de Abreu Freire. He adopted the name of Egas Moniz from a Portuguese patriot who fought the Moors. Qualified in medicine but served as Portuguese Ambassador to Spain and the Vatican, Foreign Minister and head of delegation at the signing of the Treaty of Versailles. Refused Presidency. Became Professor of Medicine in Lisbon in his middle forties. Pioneered cerebral arteriography as safer method of visualising brain outlines than Dandy's air ventriculography. Shared Nobel Prize for Medicine 1950 for introduction of prefrontal leucotomy. Retired aged 65 after being shot by psychotic patient.

Osler, Sir William (1849–1919)

Born in Canada, qualified at McGill University and became Professor of Medicine there at age of 25. Subsequently occupied chairs at Philadelphia and Johns Hopkins. Appointed Regius Professor of Medicine at Oxford 1904. His textbook *The Principles and Practice of Medicine* ran into 14 editions by 1942. A noted bibliophile, he left his library to McGill University. His interest in medical history is still commemorated in the Osler Club of London.

Paracelsus (1493–1541)

Aureolus Philippus Theophrastus Bombastus von Hohenheim. Born near Zurich, studied at University of Basle and with the Abbot of Spronheim, an alchemist. Spent time in the Tyrol studying ores, metals and minerals and the diseases of miners. An original thinker, considered to be the founder of medical chemistry. His writings are obscure and display allegorical, mystical and symbolic features.

Pavlov, Ivan Petrovitch (1849–1936)

Son of a country priest. Studied medicine at St Petersburg and did research in Breslau and Leipzig before returning there as Director of the Institute of Experimental Medicine 1891, and Professor 1897. His first work was on the circulation and the digestion. Nobel Prize for Medicine 1904. Work on conditioned reflexes in animals was followed by study of higher nervous activity in man.

Phrenology

> This is the name given to 'the new anatomy and physiology of the brain and nervous system of Drs Gall and Spurzheim' by Thomas Forster (1789–1860), a medical graduate of Cambridge, who wrote on the periodical variation of the symptoms of insanity. Franz Joseph Gall (1758–1828), MD Vienna 1785, became physician to the Establishment for the Deaf and Dumb there. He examined the heads of the inmates, of mental patients, idiots, criminals and those specially gifted, such as musicians. From this he concluded that there were special faculties with their seats in the brain and with corresponding contours on the skull. He delineated such faculties as amativeness, acquisitiveness, self-esteem etc. to the number of 27. His pupil and collaborator, Johann Gaspar Spurzheim (1776–1832) increased them to 35. Like Mesmer, Gall was forced to leave Vienna and eventually settled in Paris.
>
> Phrenology was never a system of treatment but one of personality appraisal, although Sir William Ellis at Hanwell in 1835 commended it for the guidance it gave in the choice of appropriate treatment. He examined the heads of all patients on admission but lamented that most admissions were incurable. George Eliot, the novelist, had her head shaved so that her friend Charles Bray could read her bumps.

Rush, Benjamin (1745–1813)

> Born in Pennsylvania. Graduated at Edinburgh 1768 and practised in Philadelphia. A signatory of the Declaration of Independence. Co-founder of first antislavery society. Credited with stopping yellow fever epidemic 1793 but William Cobbett in 1800 demonstrated by use of death rates that Rush's bleeding and purgation treatment was not merely useless but injurious. Considered to be Father of American Psychiatry for his *Medical Inquiries and Observations of Diseases of the Mind* 1812. His Tranquilliser was a chair in which an excited patient was immobilised.

Sakel, Manfred (1900–57)

> Qualified in medicine at University of Vienna 1925. Worked in private medical clinic (Lichterfelder Hospital) in Berlin 1927–33. Returned to Vienna as a refugee where he introduced insulin coma therapy. Again as a refugee, he went to the USA in 1937, where he gave training in insulin therapy to staff of

New York State Department of Mental Hygiene. Honoured by University of Vienna in 1957 shortly before his death.

**La Salpêtrière**

Built as an arsenal during the reign (1610–43) of Louis XIII. It became an asylum for beggars, prostitutes and the insane and it was the largest poorhouse for women. There were more than 4000 inmates in the second half of the nineteenth century.

**Tuke, William (1732–1822)**

Born into a Quaker family which had resided in York for three generations. Succeeded to the family business of wholesale tea and coffee merchants before he was 20. Founded The Retreat at York in 1792 and became its Manager and its Treasurer. The *Dictionary of National Biography* wrongly ascribes to him his grandson's description of The Retreat.

**Tuke, Samuel (1784–1857)**

Grandson of William Tuke. Like his father, Henry, he wished to become a doctor but bowed to parental wishes and entered the family business at 13. Took a great interest in insanity and the construction of asylums. In 1813 he published his *Description of The Retreat*, containing 'An account of its Origin and Progress, the Modes of Treatment and a Statement of Cases'. Was an honorary member of the Medico-Psychological Association.

**Tuke, Daniel Hack (1827–95)**

Youngest son of Samuel Tuke. His twin brother died at birth. Was apprenticed to the law but gave it up. In 1847 he started two years work as steward at The Retreat then studied at St Bartholomew's Hospital and the Royal College of Surgeons and took his MD degree at Heidelberg in 1853. He was physician to the Retreat and the York Dispensary and lectured on mental diseases at the York School of Medicine. Between 1859 and 1875 he lived at Falmouth because of ill-health. As a consultant in London he was a governor of Bethlem and lecturer in mental diseases at Charing Cross Hospital. From 1880 he edited the *Journal of Mental Science* and was President of the Medico-Psychological Association in 1881. The first edition of the *Manual of Psychological Medicine*, which he wrote with J.C. Bucknill, was published in 1858 and he was a major contributor to the Dictionary of Psychological Medicine which he edited in 1892. He was also one of the founders of the Mental After-Care Association in 1879.

Wagner-Jauregg, Julius (1857–1940)

Professor of Neurology in Graz, then in Vienna. Worked six years in Institute of General and Experimental Pathology. Published first observations in 1887. No success with inoculation of streptococci and tuberculin. First successful treatment of dementia paralytica with malaria 1917. Awarded Nobel Prize for Medicine 1925. His *bon mot* about hypnosis 'You never know who is pulling the other fellow's leg'.

Watson, John Broadus (1878–1958)

Born in South Carolina. Studied philosophy and psychology at a local Baptist college before going to Chicago. Professor of Psychology at Johns Hopkins University 1908. Taught behaviourist psychology. Forced to resign when divorced in 1920. Married his graduate assistant Rosalie Rayner. Did market research, became advertising agency executive. Advocated a scientific view of parenthood and warned against the dangers of too much mother love. Bertrand Russell thought that he had done more for psychology than anyone since Aristotle.

Willis, Thomas MD Oxon., FRCP, FRS (1621–75)

Sedleian Professor of Natural Philosophy at Oxford. His researches into the brain and nervous system made him the founder of Neurologie (his own term), and the connecting arteries at the base of the brain are named the circle of Willis. He discounted the uterus as the cause of hysteria and differentiated between organic brain disease and mental illness.

# Bibliography

There are six invaluable source books of which I have made great use:

*Three Hundred Years of Psychiatry 1535—1860*. Hunter R. and Macalpine I. (1963). Oxford: Oxford University Press.

*World History of Psychiatry*. Howells J.G., ed. (1975). London: Baillière Tindall.

*A History of Medical Psychology*. Zilboorg G. and Henry G.W. (1941). New York: W.W. Norton.

*Chapters in the History of the Insane in the British Isles*. Tuke D.H. (1882). London: Kegan Paul.

*The Historical Development of British Psychiatry*, vol. 1 *18th and 19th centuries*. Leigh D. (1961). Oxford and London: Pergamon Press.

*The Compact Edition of The Dictionary of National Biography* (1975). Oxford: Oxford University Press.

# Index